THE RAW SECRETS

THE RAW VEGAN DIET IN THE REAL WORLD

BY FRÉDÉRIC PATENAUDE
EDITOR OF *JUST EAT AN APPLE* MAGAZINE

Raw Vegan
Montreal, Canada
2002

DISCLAIMER

The responsibility for the consequences of your use of any suggestions or procedures described hereafter lies not with the authors, publisher or distributors of this book. This book is not intended as medical advice.

Editor: Andrew Durham
Cover art: Martin Mailloux

First Edition, October, 2002
Printed in Canada
ISBN 0-9730930-0-5

If you would like to publish sections of this book, please contact the publisher.

PUBLISHED BY:

Raw Vegan
6595 St-Hubert, CP 59053
Montreal (Quebec)
H2S 3P5, Canada
www.rawvegan.com
info@rawvegan.com

CONTENTS

AKNOWLEDGMENTS

Special thanks to **Albert Mosséri,** for letting me translate his writings. Without his knowledge, this work would not have been possible.

Special thanks to **Andrew Durham,** for his insights which have helped clarify many areas of this book, and for his constant support in this project and everything else.

I would like to thank all the people who have directly or indirectly contributed to the realization of this book:

Marianne Moineau — for your constant support and belief in this project; our long conversations and experiments that have helped formulate my thoughts and ideas; and your help in the realization of this project.
Olivier Magnan — for the initial motivation and idea that led to the creation of this book. C'était ton idée!
Fabi Reaume — for much-needed proofreading.
Beata Barinbaum— for your last minute critique of the book and proofreading.
Robert Harrison — for your help in proof-reading the book.
The Boutenko Family — for some last minute, raw inspiration! Спасибо!

David Norman — for your support through the years of all of my endeavors.
Enrique Candioti — for the raw inspiration and your help with the magazine.

Nature's First Law — for resuscitating this movement and providing the initial drive for all of us to really *do this.*
Paul Nison — whose rational approach to the raw diet has helped me formulate many areas of this book.
Dr. Doug Graham — whose research has helped clarify my thinking in many areas of this book.
Dr. Fred Bisci — whose insights have helped me formulate some areas of this book.

Louiselle Houle— pour avoir procuré un endroit où rester durant les débuts de ce project.
Réal Patenaude — qui m'a toujours encouragé dans mes projets.
Sébastien Patenaude — for being part of my first raw experiences and the support (ça aide d'avoir un frère).

Foreword

INTO THE DEPTHS

by Andrew Durham

Like my friend, Frédéric, I have inquired into the mystery of diet for a long time. Early on, I came across raw eating, and, like many of you, it immediately appealed to me. Always on my mind, it has swung between obsession and low-level interest.

Frédéric helped me make my first transition to an extended, raw diet. In ways he describes in this book, my experience was… not entirely pleasant. After 18 months, and feeling worse than I ever had, I bailed. In 15 years, I have never doubted the simple truth of the raw diet. I just figured I had more to learn about it and that, eventually, I'd get there.

Since then, I've found out that I bought into a lot of shallow, dietary fantasies during my early, raw days. In exposing this nonsense to myself, I have been, by turns, amused, appalled and dumbstruck: both at my misleaders and at my imbalanced, credulous approach. So helping to produce this book gratifies me for two reasons. One, it delivers a series of mortal blows to the myths and fads of popular raw eating — and my delusions about them. Two, it clears the rightful place at center stage for Natural Hygiene, which owns most of the depths of the modern, raw movement

That I might share with you my appreciation for the gravity of this project, I wish to explore depth itself for a moment and relate it back to the title of this book. Why does an approach to a subject possess depth? Because it names the subject's background issues.

Background issues form a subject's context. They hold the basic questions and premises of our inquiry into it. They give it structure, meaning and purpose. And, being little noticed, they command the allure and seductiveness of secret things.

Hunger is an example of a background issue. There would be no wonderment about diet, let alone books, without the unsettling fact of hunger. Yet almost no one discusses it (presumably because almost no one has experienced hunger, or because they fear it). Of those who do, only a few manage to remain undistracted by safe but secondary topics (like *what* to eat) and keep hunger at the center of discussion. True to the teachings of his great, hygienic instructor, Mosséri, Frédéric is learning here to hold hunger high.

Myself, I look forward to seeing the germination in this movement, from those who still carry the seed, of the ancient, German grasp of the *social* background of natural diet (see *Children of the Sun* by Gordon Kennedy). Then we'll see what radical raw eaters — a circling tribe — look like. Then, in response to their animal ensemble, we'll each feel the depth I'm talking about pulsing in our bodies. The lone harbingers of that once-and-future tribal way of life only foreshadow it now. But in darkness, they gather to tell the old stories and beat on immutable drums.

Depth calls those who are quiet enough to hear it to peer into that darkness and to discern the background issues. In our age, the darkness (fog by day) surrounds so many of us that its general examination would seem natural. Yet we can count on few to do so, for it entails committing the great crime of *slowing down*. They alone find out these crucial, fundamental things we call *secrets*. These people see what others will not even look at, precisely because of its ubiquity. Thus, the secret has become synonymous with the obvious. I'm not saying it is loud, just that it is plain.

I have sat with many who preferred the plain to the glamorous. It is my pleasure to keep finding myself next to the fire with Frédéric Patenaude. For one thing, he's a riot. For another, he always has a drop of water when I burn myself (thanks). And he takes pleasure in naming background issues, those of diet in particular. Even more rarely, he can integrate them into a principled grasp and presentation of the subject.

So what have I told you here? Just that secrets, depth, darkness and stillness go hand in hand. That there is something potent you can know about this stuff for yourself. That you will have to stare at it awhile before you even see it. And that, when you do, it will stop you in your tracks, then move you onto a bright, new course, like the sun after a pole shift.

I believe *The Raw Secrets* will challenge you as no book has since *Nature's First Law* lit a fire under the raw movement. In the debris field it has become, this book clears a wide swath. The book's ideas excite and disturb. You might even find yourself helping to clean up (for it will take many of us). Please record your experiences. We'd be thrilled to consider their inclusion in future editions.

If you have ever stopped to wonder *Why?* about anything dietary, this book is for you. If the decadence of popular veganism or raw eating has got you down, read on. If you've lost interest in marching with our culture to the abyss and would rather just live, you've come to the right place. If the battery in your bullshit meter has died, settle in for a recharge. And if you are a huckster, take cover. I give you my friend and comrade, the always colorful Frédéric, from the hip.

Andrew Durham, editor
October, 2002
Montreal, Quebec, Canada

Introduction

IN THE RAW

Radical ideas have much more power than common advice. But in their power lies danger. Like an explosive charge, radical ideas must be handled carefully.

The raw vegan diet is such an idea. It can save your life. It can banish "incurable" conditions. It can help you feel great all the time. It can give back your joy of living. It can give an entirely different direction to your life or turn it upside down. But its practical application may be difficult. Pitfalls line the path of raw eating. Many people have fallen into them — and they will continue falling into them — until they know what these pitfalls are and how to spot them.

Some people are damaging their health by eating the raw diet incorrectly. Mostly, this is because they received poor or confusing advice. This book is my antidote to the false information that is being spread in the raw food movement, hurting people as it goes. This is the book I wish someone had handed to me six years ago when I started out on this path. I intend it not as an introductory book on the subject, but rather, as a book for those who have some knowledge of and interest in the raw diet.

My dietary adventures have led me to write *The Raw Secrets*. Even though I had recognized the truth of raw-foodism at once, my personal experience with it has not been an instant success story. It has been the most positive thing I have ever done — and it has also been a struggle. Before revealing my findings, I wish to share with you here my story.

I became aware of the link between diet and health at the age of 16, when my mother introduced vegetarianism into my family. She had decided to make some changes in her diet in order to lose some weight. Suddenly, whole wheat bread, tofu, seitan and other strange items made their appearance in our fridge. Meat slowly disappeared.

Mom's interest in nutrition quickly spread to me as I started to read the books on the subject that she had bought. I slowly became a vegetarian without calling myself one. A couple years later, the final blow came when I read the book *Diet For a New America* by John Robbins, which definitely convinced me to become a vegetarian and gave me all the right reasons to do so.

Vegetarianism was fun to me. I remember the excitement of discovering all these new products; of shopping at health food stores for the first time; of learning to make new foods; and of trying to impose my new beliefs on friends and family at the first opportunity. It was fun. But vegetarianism didn't turn my world upside down.

Raw-foodism did.

By chance I found a little book by Herbert Shelton, called *Food Combining Made Easy*. It made a strong impression on me. Shelton stated that humans, like other frugivorous animals on the planet, are meant to live on fruits, vegetables, nuts, and seeds — and nothing else. For a grain-based vegetarian, this statement drilled a big hole into my comfortable, newly found, vegetarian box. I thought I had found the ultimate diet. But here came this guy saying that not only I would have to give up meat and dairy, but also grains, beans, oils, salt, seasonings, as well as everything cooked and processed! I felt assaulted and thought that I had to find out more about this stuff, because it couldn't possibly be right.

On the same shelf as Shelton's works, I came across some strange-looking books in French by a guy named Albert Mosséri. I was shocked to discover that he was saying the same things. Our natural diet should be composed of fruits and vegetables, and maybe some nuts and seeds. But more than these matters of content and instruction, these books on Natural Hygiene were saying that each of us is solely responsible for his or her health. That all the sickness that we experience is the result of wrong living — primarily the wrong diet. And that by returning to a simple, raw diet of fruits and vegetables and by fasting, we could not only heal from all these diseases, but we could also go back to our pristine, natural state, which is nothing less than exuberant health.

So I kept reading more about Natural Hygiene. I remember the feelings I had looking at the photo on the cover of Mosséri's book. In the photo there was a bowl of fruit, a few chestnuts, and a strange looking squash. It seemed so austere, yet, so attractive. And so true. I remember the conflict that was going on inside of me. "I know this is for real. What these people are saying makes a lot of sense. But then to actually do this requires that I change my life around and make it go in a completely different direction than what I had thought." That's what a 20 year-old guy was going through somewhere in Quebec, Canada. And I thought I was all alone.

So I did this on my own and without much success. I kept going back and forth. My diet was chaotic, and too much had been stirred up inside of me that I didn't know what to do with. I needed to meet some new people, to get the hell out of Canada and find out what was going on elsewhere. So one night on the Internet I found out about a book called *Nature's First Law: The Raw Food Diet*, by Arlin, Dini, and Wolfe.

Like everybody who responds positively to *Nature's First Law*, it seriously motivated me to go all-raw. I got in contact with the authors in San Diego and arranged for a meeting. I went all-raw for six months in Canada, got a couple friends into it, and worked to save money at the same time. Then I packed up my stuff and, needing to take my time to absorb all of this, boarded a 72-hour, six-layover bus to California.

In California I found the raw-food movement fresh and young, but also confused and full of contradiction. I found myself going along with the wave, being part of what was happening. Somehow along the way I got the idea that the raw diet was the answer to everything. That it would not only solve all of my problems, but it would also solve all of humanity's problems. Perhaps this enthusiasm has been necessary to get me, and all of us, started, but it certainly misled me and many others.

In California, although I was trying to maintain an air of balance and enthusiasm, my health was going slowly downhill. Too bad for a young guy like me. I found that I was constantly running out of energy. Many I felt spacy, unable to concentrate, and unable to find the energy needed to go on with normal, daily activities. I thought I was going through a detox and that this would stop one day, that I would finally feel "paradise health." Unfortunately, that day never came. The "detox" was never-ending.

Behind the scenes, seeds and fats were taking over my diet. I was sometimes eating 5-6 avocados a day as well as a lot of nuts and seeds. I started using oil, condiments, salt, garlic, and other foods that, while following Natural Hygiene in Canada, I had eschewed. I had begun to eat to pacify my cravings. Since the last thing I wanted to do was eat cooked food, I created all sorts of replacements for the cooked foods I was craving. I went berserk with raw food recipes: raw pies, raw chocolate, raw lasagna, you name it. All-raw. All organic. All healthy... right? But...

After a year, I got really sick for an entire month. But I told almost nobody because I was a raw-foodist and I was supposed to be healthy. I wasn't supposed to get sick like that. So I hid at home and fasted. After that, things became clearer. I realized that the raw diet couldn't be done haphazardly. I was still clueless about how to do it. Excluding nuts from my diet for a while after the fast really helped, but I was still far from "paradise health." Where was the boundless energy to dance all night? Where had the fire gone?

To top it off, I was this guy working at *Nature's First Law*, "world headquarters for the raw food diet." There, I had started my own raw newsletter, *Just Eat An Apple*, and I was on my way to writing a recipe book, having become quite a good raw chef.

This may all sound very dramatic. I must say that I felt like that only some of the time. I wasn't always drained, but for a big chunk of my time as a strict raw-foodist in California, I was trying to figure out why this wasn't *really* working for me, the way it was supposed to, according to the books. And I was not alone. I was meeting a lot of other people going through the same thing. But clouded by the ideal of raw-foodism, we wouldn't admit to ourselves what was going on.

When I moved back to Canada in 2000, I'd had it. I started eating cooked food again, and dammit, I started feeling better. I started feeling better because I had stepped back from my *position* of being a strict raw-foodist and was able to see the raw food diet for what it was. I saw it as a tool, one that could be used poorly, or one that could be used properly. I just hadn't learned how to use it properly yet.

Because I am given to excessiveness, I re-explored the cooked diet just as fully as I had explored the raw diet. Slowly and carefully, I tested cooked food on my body. I tried bread. I tried cheese. On dates at restaurants, I drank wine. I felt what it is like to order a croissant in a café in Paris. After a little while, I realized that I had changed my body so much by eating a raw diet that I could no longer eat the stuff I used and feel "normal" like "normal people." I needed to find something, and fast, because I knew that eating like this wasn't for me.

Back at square one. I rediscovered Natural Hygiene. I carefully reread Mosséri's books. The ones I had been reading before going to California. The books that had turned my life upside down and gave me the courage to go live somewhere else for two and a half years with only $600 in my bank account.

The rediscovery of Natural Hygiene has been very powerful for me. Having gathered all that experience, I could fully grasp the basic principles of health delineated by Hygiene. I could see them at work in everything that had happened to me and others. I was able to see what had gone wrong for me and why. Through this new understanding, I was able to go back to the diet of fruits, vegetables, nuts and seeds — which I had always wanted to eat — and actually thrive on it.

To get back to the raw diet, I had to start with small steps. First, I found that the most important thing was to limit myself to the foods which are biologically specific to human beings: fruits, vegetables, and *small* quantities of nuts and seeds; and to avoid grains, beans and condiments. I had to pay attention to hunger, food combinations, and the quantities of fat, nuts and seeds in my diet. I found that when eating baked roots or steamed vegetables, I felt much better than when I was eating lots of nuts and seeds or complicated raw recipes.

Since the all raw diet is the one that attracted me in the first place, I eventually found my way back to it. And this book is the sum of the steps that I took in order to do that. Each chapter contains a lesson, a message to myself about the subject that helped me see the whole picture again. Some of the chapters are combative, reflecting the struggles I went through. Some are more positive, reflecting the insights that occurred to me.

I understood that the raw diet is not so simple to put in practice. You can very easily damage your health eating a raw diet, probably without being aware of it at first.

My main problem for many years was the lack of energy . I often felt drained, even though I was eating the best foods in the world. It took me a long time to figure out what was going on. Unfortunately, the only advice I received from raw-foodists was, "Keep on eating raw until you get through the detox."

I have met all sorts of people doing this diet, from the sensible to the fanatical and everything in-between. Some of them looked really healthy, while others looked like they had just escaped from a death camp. I met some people who ate what they called a raw diet for many years and then went back to bread and meat. Others who had sworn in the name of Raw that they'd never go back to cooked eating were latter found enjoying hot bean burritos without a sign of guilt. How did this happen?

Balanced people tend to quickly figure this out on their own. For them, it takes four days to see what others like me take four years to sort out. Their reason and intuition are in good order. But imbalanced or extreme people (a lot of us) don't find it so easy, especially when our only guides are a few poorly researched and written books. Sadly, most of the books on the raw diet fit this description. Yet, people still need good guides, so I offer *The Raw Secrets*.

Just as the book, *Fit For Life*, misled people years ago, making them believe that they were practicing Natural Hygiene just because they were combining bread or chicken properly, new raw-foodists on the scene are being misled into thinking that they are eating a healthy raw diet just because the foods they eat are *unheated*.

There are plenty of ideas and talk but a lack of facts and wisdom. There is definitely a lack of basic principles. And this lack leads to major confusion. When people go to raw-food festivals, such as the Portland Festival, they come home very inspired, and some also very confused. Why? Because while all the speakers promote a raw diet, they disagree on what it consists of. One says that fruit is the best of foods, another says it feeds internal mold. One promotes a supplement, while another says that no supplements should ever be consumed. One guy recommends fasting, while the other says it is dangerous and that we should take juices instead. And so on. All this confusion exists because most raw-foodists — teachers and students alike — are unaware of the basic principles of health. The lack of basic principles in any science will lead to its disintegration. And this lack is particularly obvious in the raw food movement, whose leaders cannot agree between themselves on what constitutes the raw diet.

Nonetheless, these basic principles exist. They were rediscovered 170 years ago by the Natural Hygienists in the United States and by the members of the German back-to-nature movement. In this book, I present some of the basic principles of Natural Hygiene and how they apply to the raw diet, undermining some raw mythology along the way.

This is pretty new stuff for most of us, and we're bound to make mistakes and commit excesses, even heinous ones. But at the end of the mistakes comes a period of ordering and cleaning up. And the first part of cleaning is taking out the garbage.

For many people, raw-foodism has become a sort of religion where cooked food is evil and raw food is salvation. Many books have exaggerated the benefits offered by the raw diet and neglected practical application. Some raw-foodists even think that anything raw is better than anything cooked. They think that all they need to do is to eat raw foods and avoid cooked foods at all costs. However, as many have discovered the hard way, health and natural diet are not so simple.

An old saying tells, "Better is often the enemy of the good." In common parlance, we say someone, "can't see the forest for the trees." By trying to be too perfect, we sometimes lose our minds.

Many raw-foodists, including myself, have promoted the concept that Dr. Doug Graham calls the Raw/Not Raw Philosophy. It is an oversimplification of all health principles into one criterion: "Is this raw?" Rather than wondering, "Is this healthy for me?" or, "What do I experience in my body after eating this," some raw-foodists only want to know, "Is this raw?" For vegans, the question is: "Is it vegan?

An adherent of the Raw/Not Raw philosophy will shun steamed vegetables, but will not hesitate to eat a jar of raw almond butter in a week, or even in a day. He will not touch anything cooked, without thinking that the way he eats could be not as healthy as some cooked diets. A convinced vegan will avoid all animal products, but he or she might use salt, sugar, processed foods out of a factory, as long as they are "vegan."

Natural nutrition asks fer more clarity. Raw-foodism is not a religion. How you eat should be based on hunger, instinct and rational principles of physiology, not an over-simplified mantra.

Raw-foodism and veganism are valid. But not the way they are sometimes practiced, especially these days. You will learn in this book how to eat a raw vegan diet in a way that is sustainable and vitalizing.

Frédéric Patenaude
October, 2002
Montreal, Quebec, Canada

1

HOW TO DETERMINE OUR NATURAL DIET

In trying to determine the best diet for us, we inevitably face the question: what is the natural diet of humans? How are we meant to eat? What foods are biologically specific to the human body?

THE ANTHROPOLOGICAL APPROACH

Many authors have tried to determine the natural diet of humans by studying the eating behaviors of our distant cousins, the great apes, and also from what little we know of the diet that was eaten by humans long, long ago. But the mystery persists, and it is unlikely that it will ever be entirely solved.

Early Hygienists acknowledged the Darwinian similarity between humans and gorillas, chimpanzees and orangutans. They reasoned that we could get clues to our natural diet from studying the primates' diets. They read the works of the time on the subject and thought they had found the answer. Everywhere in these books, it was claimed that the great apes live on fruits and nuts alone. From there came the idea that the fruitarian diet was the most natural for us.

But this turned out to be quite mistaken. Subsequent researchers have found that: gorillas ate no nuts and hardly any fruit; chimpanzees ate a lot of fruit, nuts, some green leaves, and sometimes, even meat; and orangutans, in addition to fruit and nuts, ate some insects. Let's take a closer look at the diet of these primates.

Gorillas — The mountain gorillas eat primarily green vegetation (95%), partly because they don't find much else in their environment. They eat rare fruits in season. According to Dr. George Schaller, a very serious researcher in this field, and also Dian Fossey, another great primatologist, they do not eat any animal products. Experiments were conducted at the San Diego Zoo where the gorillas where given the choice between fruit and greens. The results were very interesting. The gorillas in the experiment ended up eating only fruit for the duration of the three months of the experiment. But I don't know if that is long enough to draw a conclusion on the frugivorous nature of these creatures.

Chimpanzees — Eat mostly fruit, some green leaves and nuts and sometimes meat. Animal products represent less than 5% of their diet.

Orangutans — Eat mostly fruit, some greens, and some nuts. When fruit is rare or not available, they eat more green leaves and some insects. Animal products represent an insignificant portion of their diet. These animals enjoy a wide variety of sweet, delicious fruits, such as rambutan, wild fig and cempedak. They are especially fond of durian.

It has been difficult to get an idea of what the ideal food of humans is based on the diets of primates, partly because these eating patterns vary greatly from one type of primate to another and even from tribe to tribe. However, we do know that they all eat a fruit-based diet, except for the gorilla, who, apparently, would like to. And they all eat greens in significant quantities. The animal products in their diet are of insignificant quantities.

Obviously we have similarities with them, so our natural diet should have similarities, but we are not exactly like them, so our diet cannot be exactly like theirs. Note that when chimpanzees eat meat, they can hunt down the animal with their bare hands and eat it freshly killed. Which one of my readers could do the same? Our living conditions are also quite different: they have access to 100% wild food, while we mostly have access to commercial, hybridized food.

HOW TO FIND THE IDEAL DIET

Mosséri quotes another hygienist:

> During the years I spent in Central America and in Cuba, I had the opportunity to observe the reaction of monkeys when offered a food they never ate before. Instinctively, they use three senses to know if the food is poisoning.
>
> • The sense of sight
> • The sense of smell
> • The sense of taste
>
> First they attentively look at the new food. If it passes this first exam of the sense of sight, they pursue their examination with their acute sense of smell. They bring their nose close to this new food and smell it intensely. If they find it has a pleasant smell, it will have passed this part of the inspection. Finally, they lick the food and taste a small piece of it. If they like the taste, they start to eat it carefully.
>
> During this whole process, the animal acted according to the *Universal Law of Natural Dietetics*, that is, they found the new food to be:
>
> • pleasant to the sight
> • pleasant to the smell
> • pleasant to the taste
>
> when it is consumed:
>
> • in the raw state
> • without combinations
> • and without seasonings
>
> This law is known by all animals, who obey it... all except man.
>
> Theofilio de la Torre
> As quoted by Mosséri in *La Nourriture Idéale*.

To this description by de la Torre, a natural hygienist of the 19th century, let us add that through the process of civilization, humans have lost much of this instinct. They cannot rely on it entirely (the mistake of instinctotherapy). Everyone, more or less, has a debased instinct.

For this reason, T.C. Fry preferred to rely on the <u>pure instinct</u> of <u>children to</u> determine our natural diet. He would imagine a table filled with all sorts of foods: fruits, vegetables, living rabbits, fish, nuts, seeds, etc., and would ask: which would a child choose? This is how he was led to believe that our natural diet was a fruitarian diet, because a child would choose fruit in preference to all other natural, raw foods.

But note that children can have a debased instinct, too — it is affected by what the mother ate during pregnancy and lactation. So in the end, it is difficult to determine the natural diet with this method. However, we can rely on our observations of biology and the knowledge accumulated during the past two hundred years by hygienists to declare that our natural diet should mainly, if not entirely, be composed of raw fruits and vegetables, with small quantities of nuts and seeds.

2

FAT

OUR FAT NEEDS

Your body doesn't need to eat fat to make fat. It can create its own fat from the other non-fatty foods that you eat. A natural diet of fruits and vegetables, with some nuts and seeds or avocado, provides essential fatty acids in sufficient quantities. Some "experts" on the subject have greatly exaggerated their benefits in order to sell their special, expensive oils. Even green vegetables contain fatty acids. Have you ever munched a bunch of plain lettuce and noticed how oily it was? There is about 1% fat in lettuce. Even fruit contains a small quantity of fat. Avocados, natural olives, and small quantities of nuts and seeds also provide us with all the essential fatty acids we could ever need. There is absolutely no need to add oil — a fractured, over-concentrated form of fat — to the diet.

Because of its complexity, fatty foods, along with protein, are the most difficult foods to digest. It has been shown that a drop of oil retards digestion for two hours. Some fat is necessary, but too much, even in a whole food like avocado, will make you tired and toxic.

You have to get your fuel somewhere. Fat is a concentrated source of it, but it also takes lots of energy to digest and it is acid-forming. On the other hand, fruit is easy to digest, provides rapid energy, and is alkaline-forming. Dr. Doug Graham pulls the covers on the situation.

"The SAD is, on average, comprised of about 42% fat. Many people on this diet eat over 50%, even 60%, of their total calories as fat. They have learned to satisfy their appetite with fats. This is not what our physiology is designed to thrive on, however. A diet dominated by the simple carbohydrates found in fruit more closely matches our physiological needs. But when going raw, most people continue consuming the high-fat diet. As they eat more vegetables, they get hungrier and eat even more fat to satisfy themselves. The simple carbohydrate deficit accrues with almost every meal.

When prospective raw-foodists go off their raw regimen, they almost invariably find themselves eating cooked, complex carbohydrates. Until they learn to consume high amounts of sweet fruits to fulfill their carbohydrate needs, they will invariably fail in their health and raw-food efforts.

The high-fat, raw-food diet is a recipe for failure, both in regards to health and to staying all raw. Utilizing the high-fruit diet is the ideal, logical and healthful method for achieving the low-fat, high-carb diet that every health practitioner on the planet recommends."

Dr. Doug Graham

ADDICTION TO FAT?

Many raw-foodists are addicted to fatty foods like nuts and seeds because they do not eat enough calories, and because they are used to eating heavy, cooked, fatty meals. They may have problems with the "detox" that never ends (see chapter 7). They feel tired all the time and blame it on detoxification. I felt like that for a long time. At some point they are convinced that raw supplements will correct this. So are they really thriving on their diet? Why not take an honest look at the diet? Someone eats five medium to large avocados a day. A single avocado usually weighs 300 grams (fruit flesh), so that's 1500 grams of avocado flesh. At 18% fat, that's 270 grams of fat, so the equivalent of over a cup of oil. What would be the consequences if you were to sit down and eat these 16 tablespoons (or 48 teaspoons) of oils?

GUIDELINES FOR EATING FATS

Unless you simply dislike them, I do not recommend avoiding avocados and nuts. You can eat them regularly with benefit. The following guidelines will help you in doing so:

• Evening is the best time to eat fatty foods. Avoid fats during the day, because they are difficult to digest and will usually make you tired. Some people can add avocado to a salad at noon.

• When eating seeds or nuts, limit yourself to 1-2 oz/30-60 g (about 15-30 small almonds). Even go so far as to get a small scale and weigh the nuts to actually know what you are consuming.

• A medium avocado weighs about 300 g. We should eat them in reasonable quantities: 2-3 avocados for athletes, 1-2 for most people, 1/2 for older folks, sedentary people and children.

• For nuts to digest, they have to be eaten on an empty stomach, not after a big salad. Eat the nuts first and then have your vegetables. Protein digests in an acidic environment, provided by the hydrochloric acid in the stomach. This is also the reason why nuts digest better when eaten at the same time with tomatoes than with greens. If you eat, for example, a big salad of cucumbers and greens, you will dilute the hydrochloric acid in the stomach. It won't be strong enough to deal with a handful of nuts you eat after, so they will just stay there and putrefy. But if you eat the nuts with tomatoes first and then the vegetables, you won't have any problems.

• Avoid the sweet fruit and fat combination. If you just eat an apple, it will digest quite fast and leave the stomach rapidly. But eat an avocado at the same time and digestion will be prolonged. The sweet fruit will have time to ferment and produce acids. The same happens when we mix nuts with dried fruits — an abominable combination that is likely to putrefy and ferment, unless it is consumed in very small quantities, such as five almonds with five dates.

• You can use some olive oil or other cold-pressed oils on your salads, but not all the time. I recommend this for beginners, but at some point, abandon this practice. It slows down digestion considerably. Those wanting more energy should avoid adding oil to their food.

• Eat one type of fatty food a day. For example, eat avocados and nuts on different days. Also, eat only one kind of nut or seed in a day.

• Desalt olives before eating them. First, remove the pits, then soak them in water for 12-24 hours, changing the water a few times in that period.

• Once or twice a month, go a few days without fatty foods.

• You can avoid fats entirely for weeks during hot weather, when the body calls for water-rich foods, such as tomatoes, cucumbers, melons, peaches, etc.

3

PROTEIN

Based on a series of articles I wrote for Get Fresh! *Magazine.*

Everyone knows that we require a certain quantity of protein every day to remain healthy. Because of propaganda to this effect, a lot of people view the daily consumption of high-protein foods like meat and dairy as beneficial. The greatest fear of the new vegetarian or raw-foodist is lack of protein. Vegetarians replace meat protein with tofu, cheese, beans and meat substitutes, while raw-foodists prefer nuts and seeds.

The opinions of experts with regard to our daily protein needs vary incredibly — from 25 to 200 grams! An average figure is 1 gram per kilogram of body weight. On a raw diet, it would be difficult to consume that much unless we ate nuts and seeds in large quantities. But judging from the failure raw-foodists are experiencing with nuts and seeds in general, it may be time to revise our ideas about protein.

SOME PEOPLE LIVE ON VERY SMALL AMOUNTS OF PROTEIN

During an expedition in the interior regions of New Guinea, the researchers Hipsley and Clements of Sidney discovered an aboriginal tribe living in the mountains of Mount Hagen whose diet consisted mainly of certain plants, 80% to 90% of their diet was sweet potatoes. The rest was composed mostly of young shoots, sugar cane, green vegetables, bananas, palm hearts and various nuts...The population, including the children and teenagers, was obviously in very good health, while accomplishing great physical work.

Professor H.A.P. Oomen... discovered that their daily consumption of protein was 9.92 grams (due to the fact that sweet potatoes only contain between 0.5 and 1.5% protein). Meanwhile they eliminated in their fecal matter around 15 times more protein than was ingested through their diet, eating between 1.4 and 2 kilos of sweet potatoes a day. The logical conclusion was that proteins were synthesized in the body following an unknown process. *biological transmutation*

Albert Mosséri
La Nourriture Idéale

Since a tribe can live on 10 grams of protein a day, it means that all theories about protein are erroneous. Also note that these people are eating a diet composed of 80 to 90% *cooked* potatoes and are in excellent health. But no group of people eating a diet composed of 80 to 90% *cooked* grains was ever found in good health.

There are other cultures in which people live on root-based diets and obtain, on average, less than 20 g of protein a day, while remaining in great health. T.C. Fry mentions the Caribs who live in the Caribbean Islands and eat a manioc-based diet and get, on average, 12 g of protein a day. They are in excellent health. The Max Planck Institute proved that, considering the fact that the body recycles most of its protein for its own needs, 25 g of protein a day is more than enough. However, most vegetarians are still terrified of not getting enough protein. As soon as they feel a lack of energy, they think to themselves, "Could it be a lack of protein?" But what about the strength of the gorilla who lives on green leaves, without the concentrated protein found in nuts?

The milk argument also easily proves that we don't need much protein. Mother's milk is, for a time, our perfect food. Only fruits and vegetables resemble it in their composition. The protein content of mother's milk is adapted to the baby's protein needs, and it *decreases* along with them. Five days after birth, protein content in mother's milk is about 2%. After seven or eight weeks, it is only 1.2%, when the baby is doubling its weight every six months.

PROTEIN IN GREEN LEAVES

Most people would not consider a salad a good source of protein. They are not aware that the protein in green leaves is of extremely high quality, containing all essential amino acids. Green leaves also contain a small, but not negligible, quantity of essential fatty acids. Although the protein content is only around 1% by weight, these proteins are highly absorbable and will not ferment in the intestines, nor will they poison the body. Green vegetables contain a lot of alkaline minerals, which help to assimilate those proteins.

Fruit, on the other end, contains a small quantity of protein (around 0.5% by weight), but this, also, is of high quality and is highly assimilable. Some of the fruits containing higher quantities of protein are: avocados (2.1%), dates (2%), bananas (1%), figs (1.5%), cherries (1%).

A raw-food diet containing small amounts of nuts and seeds provides about 25-35 grams of protein a day, which is about what the Max Planck Institute recommends, and consequently, more than what the tribes mentioned were eating. This quantity is also what gorillas eat. And still, many authors recommend eating too much protein. Excess protein is actually dangerous, whether it comes from meat or from plant sources. Like fat, it is extremely complex and difficult to digest. It is acidifying and so leaches alkaline minerals out of the body to balance pH.

DISEASES AND CONDITIONS CAUSED OR AGGRAVATED BY EXCESSIVE PROTEIN CONSUMPTION
by Albert Mosséri

- Infection
- Pus
- Abcess
- Fever
- Cancer

- Kidney disorders
- Leukemia
- Impaired vision
- Fistulas, boils, urticaria
- Skin diseases

- Number of people in America suffering from diseases caused by protein excess: 40,000,000
- Number of people in America suffering from diseases caused by protein deficiency: 3

(From *Diet for a New America* by John Robbins)

We should not worry about getting insufficient protein. As long as we eat, we will get enough. *We should worry about getting too much of it.* If we eat enough green vegetables and fruits to meet our needs (2 to 3 kilos, or 4-6 pounds, of food a day for most people), we will not *exceed* our protein needs.

4

NUTS AND SEEDS

Based on a series of articles I wrote on nuts and seeds for Get Fresh!

THE DIET OF PRIMATES, OR, HOW TO KNOW WHAT TO EAT

The first authors to write about raw-foodism and natural hygiene tried to find out what constituted the ideal human diet. To find an answer to this knotty puzzle, they studied the diet of primates, declared by science to be our "closest relative," thus hoping to find in the regimen of these hairy creatures the most appropriate menu for humans wishing to conform to the laws of Nature (with a capital N!). But in view of the fact that the great apes were getting rare and the costs and difficulties of travel were very high, paying them a visit in the heart of the jungle was not a practical solution. Instead, they examined the few zoological studies existing at the time.

Somewhere in those books, someone said that the great apes lived on fruits, vegetables, nuts and seeds. This affirmation didn't stun our budding rawists. Aren't these foods the most pleasing to the palate when eaten in the raw state? All the rest (grains, dairy, meat, etc.) has to be seasoned and cooked to be appreciated. On the other hand, fruits, vegetables, nuts and seeds, can be eaten with delight without any seasoning or cooking.

It is by using this reasoning that early vegetarians, natural hygienists, and raw-foodists claimed everywhere that fruits, vegetables, nuts and seeds, consumed in their raw state, constituted the natural diet of humans.

But since then, many things have changed. To confuse the picture, we have learned that gorillas eat mostly greens, almost no fruit and no nuts or seeds. Orangutans, on the other hand, eat mostly only fruit, very few nuts and some greens. And then there are the chimpanzees, who, in addition to nuts and greens, eat a lot of fruit and some have even been caught eating meat!

PROBLEMS FROM EXCESSIVE NUT CONSUMPTION

Some authors have started to question the value of nuts in the raw-food diet. They have done this not by scientific reasoning, but after noticing the effects of nuts on themselves and their patients.

But there have always been those in favor of nuts, essentially because they are the only protein-rich foods in the raw vegetarian diet. Because protein deficiency has frightened us, we take comfort in the daily consumption of nuts.

Herbert Shelton recommended around 100 to 120 grams of nuts a day, which is about a large handful of almonds (around 50-70 almonds). But few people are able to digest this quantity of nuts everyday. The French natural hygienist, Albert Mosséri, wrote:

> I observed innumerable problems and even serious accidents following such a consumption of nuts: liver problems, skin disorders, dizziness, fatigue, lowering of the digestive powers, urinary infection, pus, smelly and abundant urine, lowered vision, myopia, sensitivity to cold, sensitivity to sun baths and light, spaciness, frequent gases, etc. I understood at once that Shelton, for all his genius and for all the admiration and respect I had for him for years, had committed, in this matter, a terrible mistake.
>
> *La Nourriture Idéale*

Following the guidelines provided in chapter 2, it is possible to eat nuts without running into these problems.

The stimulation from overeating nuts is comparable to the stimulation people get from eating meat. When we overload the system with this excess protein, the body "fights" in response to it, and it is this fight for life, in other words, this stimulation that we perceive as energy. Again, it is an illusion, just like the false energy people get from coffee, sugar, or chocolate. This so-called energy is just the heightened activity of the body fighting to reject the excess poison.

We have to understand the following: it's not the protein in nuts that is dangerous, but the *excess* protein that putrefies and ferments in the intestines, poisoning the whole body. Thinking that we need excessive amounts of protein is what actually compromises our health. A smaller quantity of highly-assimilable protein would fill our small needs much better.

IN NATURE

Raw-foodists like to talk about what is natural versus what is not. So what is the place of nuts in the natural diet of humans? The first thing that I realized when rethinking this was that nuts are a seasonal food. They are not fresh all year round, but only 2-3 months out of every year. Then I found that there was a major difference between a fresh raw nut and a dried one. Dried nuts fill us more because, having lost most of their living water, their fat and protein concentration is higher. But is it natural to eat nuts this way?

When I was in Spain I had the occasion to taste fresh almonds straight from the tree. It was an extremely satisfying treat — crunchy, creamy, and still watery, but with a certain fat content. I thought, wow, this is how we're supposed to eat nuts.

Those who like to compare us to the other frugivorous animals will find it interesting to study the diet of the apes. Most of them live mainly on fruits and green leaves and will eat nuts when they are in season a few months a year. The gorillas do not eat any nuts and are the biggest and strongest of all. They eat the human equivalent of 25-30 grams of protein a day (if we do the math and relate this to our weight in comparison to theirs). Orangutans seldom eat nuts, and then only when they can find them. Chimpanzees are the biggest nut eaters, but they are also known for their violent behavior of attacking, killing and eating other monkeys.

THE NEEDS OF CHILDREN AND PREGNANT WOMEN

After reading one of my articles about nuts and seeds, one thoughtful person wrote to me: "I just wanted to say that your article about nuts in *Get Fresh* was very good and uplifting. Can you please expand just a little bit on the same subject concerning raising children and their needs while growing? It sounds good for adults, but how about kids and toddlers?"

Like my correspondent pointed out, my ideas on nuts and protein mainly concern adults. It is obvious that growing children have different needs than adults. However, let's review some facts first:

• Gorillas and orangutans raise their children mostly without concentrated protein with good results.
• A human baby should not receive solid food for at least one year, if not 2-3 years, living solely on mother's milk, with some soft fruits and vegetables.
• Protein content of mother's milk, and a baby's corresponding needs, starts low (relative to other mammals) and goes down from there.
• Babies cannot chew nuts properly.
• Fruits and vegetables also contain protein. Green vegetables contain high-quality protein. Avocados contain 2% protein. Dates contain 2% protein.
• If vegan children absolutely needed nuts in order to be healthy (which is not the case), this would be a proof that the vegan diet is not sufficient for children. Nuts cannot be found all year round in nature.

My recommendations are the following: you can include *some* nuts in a child's diet, but babies and children under three years of age should not have them because they are supposed to drink mother's milk. *Nut milks are acid-forming and cannot replace mother's milk.* If, for some reason, the mother cannot nurse, the baby should be given diluted, ideally raw, animal milk (preferably goat's milk).

Children can have some nuts, as long as they chew them well. Since the maximum for adults is one or two ounces (30-60 g), the same amount should suffice for children, alternated with avocados. One day the avocado, one day the nuts. But it appears more important to me that children be given enough green leafy vegetables every day to insure they get all the minerals they could possibly need. Green leafy vegetables contain the highest quality protein and an abundance of minerals. Children should get at least one large salad or blended salad a day and celery juice should be added to their fruit juices, if fruit juices are given.

Pregnant and lactating women should also eat enough green vegetables — so I advise them to eat a large salad every day or a blended salad, and one glass of vegetable juice.

It is beneficial to eat nuts in small quantities, which can be different for every individual. The maximum should be around 30-60 g, (about 15-30 small almonds) and maybe a little more for athletes and strong constitutions. But I don't think we need to eat them everyday. Eating avocados and nuts on separate days is better. We should also avoid nuts and seeds during the summer because they are not in season at that time of the year.

5

Teeth

Based on a series of articles I wrote on nuts and seeds for Get Fresh!

Until starting the raw diet, many raw-foodists, including myself, had normal dental health. Then, after a few months to a few years, dental problems appeared — lots of cavities, dental erosion and general decay. This has not happened to everyone, but to enough people to make us wonder and try to understand what has gone wrong.

Many have accused the sugar and acids in fruit. This contributes to the problem, but in my opinion, it is only a small part of it. Of course, if you eat 20 oranges a day, or drink liters of grapefruit juice, you cannot expect your teeth to last very long. There is a limit to the quantity of fruit acids the body can handle.

Cavities may be caused by constant acidity in the mouth and this acidity may be caused by acid-forming foods. Also, when the body is in a constant acidic (toxic) state, it will literally "rob" calcium from the bones The calcium is used to neutralize the acids. At least, this is one theory. Thus, the constant acidity in the mouth caused by an excess consumption of concentrated protein foods may cause tooth decay. Eating 120 grams (or more)of nuts everyday is enough to ruin the teeth of almost anyone.

Teeth and Nuts

Nothing can ruin teeth as fast as nuts and seeds. They also create tooth abscesses, like those belonging to a general infection.

However, in the long run, cavities are caused by grains, including bread and rice. 90% of children in school have cavities and adults, even more so.

Research was done on the excellent health and perfect dentition of the Polynesians. Their diet was composed of 85% starchy root vegetables. But as soon as they changed this diet and replaced their staple foods with grains, their teeth started to deteriorate early in childhood.

This shows that starch is not responsible for the deterioration, because root vegetables, like grains, contain a lot of it. It must be the protein content of the grains that leads to a demineralized body and causes cavities. In addition to this, grains contain proteins particular to seeds, so we must accuse a certain germination propensity that is antagonistic to humans. In fact, 10 grams of protein in green leaves, vegetables or potatoes do not have the same effect and do not cause the same damage as the same dose of protein in seeds.

It is true that when proteins are free of this seminal quality, as is the case with meat, the damaging effects are not as obvious, especially when meat is eaten raw with the cartilage and bones, which contain all the essential nutritive elements of the animal. This explains why vegetarians who consume nuts and seeds as well as grains experience poorer health than those who eat meat in moderation. And those who eat some meat have even better health when they refrain from eating grains and replace them with potatoes instead.

According to a dentist who emphasizes prevention, nuts and seeds have a too high potassium and phosphorus content, which robs the body of calcium, thus causing cavities and pyorrhea, if not abscess.

Albert Mosséri
La Nourriture Idéale

David Wolfe recommends eating 100 grams of green vegetables for every 10 grams of nuts in order to balance the phosphorus content (and other acid minerals) in the nuts with the calcium (and other alkaline minerals) found in green vegetables. He recommends this to avoid the acid-forming effects of the nuts. This seems easy to do when eating 20-30 grams of nuts — we can all eat a big salad containing 300 grams of green vegetables. But when eating 100 grams of nuts, who eats two or three pounds of lettuce and kale? But in reality, who would or could eat that many greens, just to balance the acidity of that many nuts? It is too much. Better to reduce the amount of nuts coming in.

6

GRAINS AND BEANS

The following is adapted from an article by Albert Mosséri.

WE ARE NOT GRANIVORES

"All true natural hygienists are opposed to grain products. These include bread, pasta, rice, flour, cookies and crackers. It seems very difficult for most people to understand this subject, because unconsciously they refuse to abandon the habit of eating bread and other grain products. "Why," they say, "it is the very foundation of civilization." Those who call themselves natural hygienists and still promote bread, even whole wheat, are not true hygienists. They don't understand that nature doesn't produce bread, that grains are meant to be eaten by birds, who are granivores (eaters of grains) and that humans are frugivores (eaters of fruit and green leaves).

"There are many reasons why grains are not suited for humans. Among the most valid are those taken from the science of biology — and consequently, are the same type of arguments that vegetarians use to condemn meat eating.

"A chart of comparative anatomy reveals that humans have none of the characteristics of the carnivore. They do not have appropriate teeth to bite the prey, nor an adequate liver to neutralize all the toxins and so on. Everybody can easily understand that humans are not carnivores. But what I say is that humans are not granivores either. We are not biologically designed to eat grains. For every class of animals on the planet, nature has provided a certain category of foods for them. Any deviation from that will create all sorts of problems: disease, cancer, psychosis, demoralization, etc.

"A machine that is supposed to function well with a certain type of oil will not function as well with a different type of oil. It will clog up and break down. This is the major argument against grains. All other "scientific" arguments are only in the details.

"Nature has provided a special type of food for fish, another type of food for cows and something entirely different for bears. And for us, nature provides us with our natural foods: fruits and vegetables. Nature is not chaotic. Every species eats the food it was designed to eat. If horses started eating meat and lions started grazing with the cow, it would be the end of everything!

THE GIZZARD

"Bread and grains, whole or not, are extremely deficient in minerals, compared to fruits and greens. They are lacking in alkaline minerals, such as calcium. Indeed, they are some of the most acid-forming foods. Our physiology is not designed to handle the digestion of grains. The ptyalin enzyme in our mouth can only handle the small amount of starch found in roots and some fruits. Species that are granivores, like some types of birds, have a special organ called the gizzard. What is a gizzard? It's a sort of second stomach that permits certain types of birds to grind hard seeds in order to digest them. With that type of strong stomach, they can even pulverize little rocks in no time. In fact, they swallow rocks to help grind grain. Even metal needles, swallowed by some young birds, are broken into pieces and rejected with no apparent damage.

"Have you ever seen chickens and other types of fowl eating rocks, nails and other hard and indigestible things? At that moment, you probably asked yourself: why are these animals eating these useless and harmful things? Have they gone mad? Or are they following their instinct? They are simply introducing hard things into their gizzard to help grind the hard seeds that they just ate.

"Birds and fowl have no teeth. That's why they have to swallow whole seeds. But since they need to digest them, Nature provides them with a perfect grinding machine attached to their stomach. Small rocks, when eaten, serve as millstones.

"But humans are much different. They do not have a gizzard. They cannot grind hard seeds like grains or legumes. This is one reason these foods are not meant for us.

"Now someone will say that we can replace the gizzard with a millstone constructed by humans, and cook the grains to soften them and render them easy to chew and digest. That's what we've been doing for several thousands of years. But this does not solve the problem._

"The digestive tract of humans and of all frugivorous animals is too long for the efficient digestion of heavy starches. These foods stay there for too long, and thus, have a tendency to ferment. Grains are natural foods for birds and fowl, but not humans. We are not equipped with a gizzard and other physiological designs in order to process grains properly.

"Furthermore, humans cannot eat and enjoy these foods in their natural state. They are simply not foods we are biologically meant to eat. Our natural foods are fruits and green leaves."

Here is Albert Mosséri's list of diseases caused by grains and bread, based on his decades of helping thousands of ill people back to health.

DISEASES AND CONDITIONS CAUSED OR AGGRAVATED BY BREAD AND GRAIN CONSUMPTION
by Albert Mosséri

- the common cold
- the flu
- sinusitis
- bronchitis
- pneumonia
- colitis
- asthma
- allergies

- respiratory
- diabetes
- arthritis
- thick blood
- arteriosclerosis
- paralysis (caused by blood clots)
- heart attacks

7

DETOXIFICATION

The great hygienist, Herbert Shelton, in his health classic, *The Science and Fine Art of Food and Nutrition*, says this about detoxification:

> Every adaptation to habits, agents and influences which are inimical to life is accomplished by changes in the tissues which are always away from the ideal. The renovating and readjusting processes that must follow a reform in living is accomplished by the tearing down and casting out of these un-ideal tissues. New and more ideal tissues take their place. The body is renewed.
>
> This process of readjustment is not always smooth. Aches and pains, loss of weight, skin eruptions, etc., may result. Helen Densmore truly says that, "If it were true that, after many years of abuse, we could stop the wrong course of living and all the blessings of health follow immediately, it would be proof that this disobedience is not so bad after all."
>
> As she says, "With the drunkard, the curative action is recognized at once — all know that it is not the water that is making him ill, but the alcoholic poison which he had been before accustomed to. So mother, sister, sweetheart and friends with one accord appeal to him to keep up his courage, notwithstanding his apparently bad symptoms. How differently is the poor dyspeptic treated when he attempts to reform his diet. With one accord his friends try to prevail on him to abandon it; assure him that he is killing himself; read him tomes of medical authorities to show that he is impoverishing his blood by his 'low diet' and when he returns to the old injurious diet, just as with the dram of spirits

in the case of the drunkard, the effect is to stop the curative action; he feels braced up and this is taken as proof that he was all wrong and the accumulation of disease commences again."

These renovating crises are seldom severe and are always followed by better health. Persistence and determination are required when they come. Most people, particularly young and vigorous ones, will make the change with very little or no discomfort.

Many of you may have heard of the concept of detoxification. When you adopt a clean diet of fruits and vegetables, the body will begin to eliminate its accumulated toxins. Since their poisonous nature is more noticeable on their way out than when they are "in storage," you will probably feel worse before you feel better. When you improve your diet, you feel a fatigue which, in fact, is just a relaxation. The body is letting go. This can take a few months — in most cases, four to eight. During this time, it is imperative to sleep more, get plenty of rest and avoid hard physical exercise and mental stress until the weight naturally starts to come back. From this point forward, you can start exercising and keep on feeding yourself properly.

THE NEVER-ENDING DETOXIFICATION

However, some people think that detoxification — the intense phase of purification — goes on forever. Years after changing their diet, they still talk about how they are "detoxifying." They attribute every headache or discomfort to the elimination of ancient debris, while ignoring their present habits. I've known long-term, "healthy" eaters who blamed their headaches on vaccines they received in their childhood!

In most cases, this intense detoxification is over within months. You will still eliminate metabolic waste for the rest of your life, but intense healing crises will occur rarely if you live in accordance with the laws of nature.

Once you stop waking up in the morning with a bad taste in your mouth, detoxification is basically over. So it doesn't make any sense to blame continuing symptoms on past mistakes. Rather, think about what you are doing now that could be draining your energy. Here are some possible causes (in no particular order):

POSSIBLE CAUSES FOR LACK OF ENERGY

- Lack of sleep
- Eating too many fatty foods, such as nuts and seeds
- Negative emotions
- Lack of or excessive exercise
- Lack of fresh air
- Lack of sunshine
- Dehydration
- Chronic stress, loneliness and anxiety
- Bad food combining
- Eating when not hungry
- Overeating
- Use of spices, salt, condiments
- Second-hand smoke

Each of these factors and many more, will drain your energies and elevate your levels of internal toxemia. When you improve your diet, you become more sensitive, so your body will let you know more quickly when there's something wrong.

THE TRUE PREVENTION

When you feel mild symptoms such as headaches, fatigue, spaciness or irritation, analyze your lifestyle and diet in the last few weeks or months and to determine what could be the reasons for your ills. Then eliminate the causes and get some extra rest. If necessary, fast for a few days on water. The hygienist, Albert Mosséri, sheds light on this subject:

> According to the Law of the Evolution of disease, examined in my book "Put Your Health into The Hands of Nature," the various diseases always begin with unnoticed signs. For example, light headaches may be felt; or a bad digestion, a lack of appetite, fatigue, a fogged and unclear mind, pessimistic ideas, bad mood, gas, constipation, vague pains here and there, etc.
>
> At the first signs of discomfort or poor health, the appropriate measures should be taken: rest, fasting, proper diet, removal of the cause. The evolution of disease is thus stopped and no complications will occur.

But if we neglect this or we suppress these first premonitory signs, by convenience — we don't want to stop working; or we prefer to suppress the symptoms with medicines to keep drinking coffee, eating meat, bread, etc. — we then stop the redeeming elimination and prepare the grounds of diseases that will afflict the person in a very precise order, going from acute to chronic.

This is how we can foresee the disease and detect it, without inefficient laboratory testing and analysis and finally obviate its harmful consequences with a simple hygienic prevention. Preventing is better than curing and it is while taking care of the first symptoms that we can prevent every disease.

Mangez Nature, Santé Nature

IT'S NOT NORMAL TO FEEL THIS WAY

After a year of eating a raw diet (or any diet) and having no serious, life-threatening health problems to start with, it is not normal to:

- Feel really tired in the afternoon
- Need to drink water during the night
- Experience many ups and downs in energy levels
- Feel worse than before you started the diet
- Feel itchiness
- Have a strong body odor
- Experience more dental problems than before
- Have regular headaches

If these conditions persist, take another look at your eating and living habits in light of the information presented in this book.

8

THE LAW OF VITAL ACCOMMODATION

The Law of Vital Accommodation is nature's wheel. The response of the vital organism to external stimuli is an instinctive one, based upon a self-preservative instinct which adapts itself to whatever influence it cannot destroy or control.

Herbert Shelton
Orthobionomics

The Law of Vital Accommodation helps clarify many dietary blind spots. This law, written in nature, states that when a poison is introduced into the organism on a regular basis, to a degree beyond the body's capacity to expel it, the body adapts to this invader by insulating itself from it. This is done at the expense of metabolic functioning. For example, if you smoke, your body will prevent absorption of the toxic fumes by hardening the lung membranes.

If you take a less than fatal dose of poison everyday, after six months you could take a more than fatal one and survive. The body will resist the poison by avoiding absorption at all cost. But this also means that general nutrient absorption will be diminished.

In *Orthobionomics*, Shelton wrote, "toleration to poisons is merely a slow method of dying. Instead of seeing in the phenomena of toleration something to be sought after, it is something to seek to avoid the necessity for."

A PURER BODY

When you begin a clean diet based on fruits and vegetables, you are no longer taking a lot of popular poisons: coffee, chocolate, cigarettes, spices, food preservatives, etc. Your body rejects accumulated poisons and goes back to a more original, pure state. In other words, you will be like the beginner before he started to take his daily dose of poison, which means that you will be much more affected by small doses of poisons than most people. A cup of coffee could have the same effect on you as five cups on your neighbor. You will be more affected by what you eat, especially if you go off your new diet. Shelton, again reiterates:

> The first smoke or the first chew of tobacco usually occasions a very powerful action against it on the part of the organism. The young man or woman is made very sick; there is headache, nausea, vomiting, loss of appetite, weakness, etc. So long as the physiological powers and instincts are undepraved and unimpaired, they instantly perceive the poisonous character of the tobacco and give the alarm to the whole system. A vigorous effort is made to destroy and eliminate it and the user is forced to throw away his tobacco. But if he continues to repeat the performance, the action against it grows less and less with each repetition, until, finally, he is able to use many times the original amount without occasioning such results. His system learns to *tolerate* it and adapt itself to its use as far as possible.
>
> *Orthobionomics*

You may think that eating a tiny bit of junk here and there might be okay: a piece of chocolate, a cup of coffee, a muffin, etc. But it will not be like the old days. Your body may violently reject the poisons each time, and these small dietary divergences may destabilize and ruin everything in the long term. Small, but regular deviations can vitiate our efforts, prevent the desired results and make one feel worse than before. This is why we have to stick to our diet as determinedly (though not fanatically) as possible. Yet, we have to distinguish the big mistakes from the small ones.

The following "foods" (drugs, really) and habits must be avoided at all times:

POISONS TO AVOID

- Coffee
- Tea
- Alcohol
- Tobacco
- Marijuana
- Drugs (legal and illegal)
- Chocolate
- Spicy food
- Junk food
- Fried foods
- Products coming from a factory
- Household chemicals (including personal care products)

9

Giving Up Bad Habits

A Popular Tendency

There is a popular tendency in the health movement that strives to do everything possible in order to appeal to the largest number of people. It assumes that most people are not ready for big changes. It assumes that they need to take baby steps, gradually and smoothly changing their habits, until they are ready to see the bigger picture. Furthermore, it assumes that most people are not ready to hear a radical message and will even frown at it.

The experts with this frame of mind not only assume that people are incapable of great changes, but also propose that people should only be encouraged to implement good habits, like eating more fruits and vegetables, rather than be discouraged to abandon bad ones, like eating meat. So they will suggest, "Eat less meat," rather than, "Become a vegetarian," which would be viewed as a move too extreme by the majority. They will propose, "Eat more fruits and vegetables," rather than, "Eliminate grain products." They will suggest, "Start juicing," rather than, "Stop smoking" or "Get more exercise," instead of, "Stop taking medications," and so on. This philosophy has its full embodiment in the saying, "An apple a day keeps the doctor away." It suggests that it does not matter how many bad habits you have, as soon as you implement new good habits, such as an apple a day, your health will improve. Eventually, the advice devolves to, "Take this supplement or drug and it will compensate for whatever bad habit you may have."

Naturopathic books are filled with such insipid recommendations, whose benefits are largely unproven and which cost little or nothing to the readers — cold showers, herbal teas, specific juices for each disease, etc. They prefer to do this rather than talk about the harmfulness of grains, coffee, chocolate, meat and dairy products. This would discourage the reader, who does not want to change his diet but only get a cure for his problems.

A man suffering from high blood pressure goes to his doctor. He smokes cigarettes, eats fried foods, meat, salt, bread and consumes almost no raw fruits and vegetables. The doctor wants to prescribe pills for him, but he won't hear of it. He goes to a naturopathic doctor. In addition to recommending a few herbal teas, the naturopath tells him that he should "think about" stopping smoking, eat "more fruits and vegetables" and "less meat." The man leaves with what he came for: a few easy excuses for not radically changing his habits. *Why not also point out the culprits instead of always hailing the saviors?*

GOOD HABITS OR BAD HABITS?

You shouldn't measure your health solely by how many good habits you have, but also by how many bad ones you have. In other words, it doesn't matter so much, however healthful it may be, that you eat "lots of fruits and vegetables," that you "juice daily," and that you," work out four times a week," if, on the other hand, you indulge in coffee, bread and meat. Your health will be directly affected by your bad habits, no matter how many good ones you have. These bad habits create illnesses. You will not get rid of them no matter how many new good habits you implement, unless you reform your lifestyle entirely.

Already I hear the voices of contention. Some people dislike this "negative" approach. Yes, it is negative. But so what — it is honest! Why not be true to facts and to yourself and thereby improve your health?

I am not saying that you shouldn't use psychology and sensitivity. Even those who are ready to reform their lifestyle are rarely capable of doing so in one day. I am not even close to suggesting such a thing. This reform should be undertaken gradually, and with an intelligent approach.

TWO APPROACHES

The *typical* advice goes like this: "You have to change your lifestyle, one piece at a time. You will slowly and gradually add more fruits and vegetables, get more exercise, daily sunshine, and you will gradually reduce your consumption of junk food, meat, dairy and pasta.

The *intelligent* advice goes like this: "You have to change your lifestyle, one piece at a time. You have several bad habits that drain your energy and are the cause of your illness. You smoke, drink coffee, eat meat, bread and cheese. Each of these habits will have to be abandoned and replaced by good habits. However, I know how difficult it is, so I will help you do it gradually. Every week or two, or at whatever rate is comfortable for you, you will *get rid* of one of these habits, until your entire lifestyle has changed. At the same time, I will teach you new healthy habits that you can start that will be both fun and interesting."

The first approach rarely has success because it disregards basic psychology. We gladly accept something to do as long as it doesn't involve getting rid of the bad habits they love. We almost never do it unless you tell them they absolutely have to (and even then). In other words, "gradually include more fruits and vegetables and exclude junk food in the diet," will be loosely interpreted. We'll grab an apple here and there, maybe order orange juice instead of a coke, and make a handful of other little changes that will hardly make a difference.

It is much easier to think about starting to juice than ceasing to drink coffee. It is basic psychology. You don't want to stop drinking coffee because it is something you like. Starting to juice is easy. But stopping a bad habit is not. It takes work and determination. The easier way is always more appealing. It's always easier to "add" than to "remove" when we talk about habits. I wish it were as easy as taking a pill, biting a few apples, and or eating some extra salad. Everyone likes to cling to their bad habits. We have to find courage to face reality and decide that — *Yes, we're going to make some real changes!*

We must also consider sources of advice and what they stand to gain. There's no money in telling people that they have to stop their bad habits in order to be healthy. There's no money in merely telling them to stop smoking. But there is in selling them a nicotine patch. There's no money in telling people to stop drinking coffee and alcohol. But there is in selling them a juicer. There's no money in telling people to stop eating fried foods, bread, meat and dairy. But there is in selling them supplements.

WHAT'S WORST?
When it comes to bad habits, there are degrees of evil. Not all habits are equally damaging. Quantities and regularity also matter. Drinking two cups of coffee a day is not the same as drinking one a month. In a rough order of importance, here are the most common bad habits that undermine health, starting with the worst ones:

- Use of drugs, prescribed and illicit
- Eating without genuine hunger; overeating
- Indulgence in chronic stress and negative emotions
- Coffee, cigarettes, alcohol, tea, chocolate and other popular poisons
- Junk foods: fried foods, fast food, factory food, etc.
- Lack of sleep
- Eating foods that are not specific to the human race: bread, grains, meat, fish, dairy products, etc.
- Using condiments, spices, salt, etc., which hinder digestion and lead to overeating
- Poor food combining
- Lack of exercise, sunshine, etc.

There are many more bad habits but I just listed the most common ones. The order may also be questionable. Several emotional states, such as depression, are caused either by medicines, by poisons contained in "fun" foods (coffee, chocolate and junk foods) and by foods in the basic diet itself (meat, fish, wheat, beans, rice and milk).

BEING EFFECTIVE
Of course people are a little better off eating more fruits and vegetables and getting more exercise. Sometimes supplementation can mitigate an abominable diet and save some people from certain

death by mineral and vitamin deficiency. But they won't get the desired results until they give up coffee, stop smoking and exclude bread, cheese, etc., from their diet. You will never "burn off" the effects of your poor diet no matter how many miles you run, how many supplements you take, or how much sunshine you get. The idea is not to try to be perfect because it is impossible. We have to take a honest look at our habits and reform our lifestyle gradually.

10

SUPPLEMENTS

SUPPLEMENTS AMONG VEGETARIANS AND RAW-FOODISTS

Supplements are as popular among vegetarians and raw-foodists, as in the general population. However, the types of supplements consumed by these two groups are different. While the average supplement consumer buys cheap vitamin and mineral supplements in hopes of "correcting" their poor diet, vegetarians and raw-foodists buy expensive, exotic, quality supplements either out of fear that their diet might be inadequate, or that the "super-health" that depends on these fancy products is the missing piece in their internal puzzle.

Super-foods and supplements abound. All are supposed to bring you exciting results. Blue-green algae, MSM, green powder, enzymes, horsetail powder, Noni fruit, Aloe Vera juice, fruit and vegetable juice powder — the list is endless. What should we think of all these products? Can they be useful or are they just another way for opportunists to fatten their wallets?

Why would raw-foodists, who are supposed to have found the most natural diet there is, need to take supplements? The supplements industry offers simple, convincing reasons, such as: The soil is of a poor quality; The fruits and vegetables we buy do not contain enough vitamins and minerals; The fruit is picked too early and has not reached maturity; and if we do not supplement, we will run into trouble. These are some of the arguments used by the supplement sellers.

If someone feels great, she could only be led to buy supplements out of fear of future deficiencies. She would have to be convinced that, although she may feel fine right now, many years from now she may run into big trouble because her diet is lacking in minerals, enzymes, vitamins or whatever. So she'd rather play it safe and take the supplement.

On the other hand, a person who doesn't feel so great can be convinced much more easily. Many become vegetarians or raw-foodists in the hope of reaching superior health. They know that they have to go through a detox period — but a few years later, still not feeling the results, they start to wonder if there is something wrong with the diet itself. Of course, they are right. There is something wrong with the way they eat, but the supplement hucksters and naturopaths are planting an entirely different doubt in their minds. They will image that they feel because their diet is lacking in whatever some supplement is "packed" with. They then proceed to spend $200 a month to buy supplements and other exotic articles. They might feel a little better, but where's "paradise-health"?

WHAT CAUSES DEFICIENCIES

In most cases, those living a natural diet do not need supplements. There are still enough vital elements in the foods you buy, as long as their taste is acceptable. And if you eat your food plain, it will be easy to detect the fake fruits and vegetables. In fact, most raw-foodists have become quite adept at selecting the best produce at hand. These fruits and vegetables may not be ideal, but *they are good enough*. Your body only needs so many vitamins and minerals and will reject the rest. If you are suffering from a deficiency, it is probably due to foods you eat that impair assimilation, not from a lack of the vital elements in them. Mosséri explains:

> Let's take the case of anemia. There is an iron deficiency in a subject. The analysis shows it. But when we scrutinize the patient's menu, we find in most cases that there is no lack of iron! In many cases, there is an abundance of iron in the diet. In fact, in pernicious anemia, there is an excess of iron-based pigments in all the internal organs. Hunter discovered that, even in fatal cases, a great quantity of iron leached from the blood could be

found in the spleen. This shows that there is more iron than is needed in the bodies of anemic people; it's just not being used.

Another proof that anemia is not caused by a lack of iron in the diet is that *this disease regresses during fasting*, while no food is eaten and no iron is provided to the body through the diet. During a short fast, we notice a marked increase in the red blood cell count. This shows that there are iron reserves in the body, but that, for some reasons, they are not used. This proves that iron found in foods and iron accumulated in the tissues have not been appropriated — assimilation is failing. This is called a faulty metabolism.

So we are not witnessing in these cases an iron deficiency in the menu, but a lack of iron absorption. This deficiency is not of an immediate dietary origin, but could be after a long time. After a seven-day fast, the red blood cell count increases noticeably. But if the fast is longer — very long — we will be sure to witness a lowering of the red blood cells count — and of many other elements — because the reserves will be used up at some point. This is why no analysis should be done for many months after breaking a fast.

In addition, when iron is prescribed in a food form, such as in artichoke extracts, no results are obtained either. What do we gain by feeding anemic people with iron-rich foods, when they already possess in their tissues abundant iron reserves, unused because they cannot be assimilated?

Albert Mosséri
Mangez Nature Santé Nature

Nearly everyone drinks milk as a calcium supplement, yet many end up suffering from osteoporosis anyway (humans cannot absorb calcium from cow's milk). No matter how much calcium they take, they will not get better until they eliminate dietary poisons that either prevent calcium absorption or leech calcium from the body. Excess protein creates acids that have to be neutralized using the body's own reserves of calcium. In this example, eating protein foods in excess (such as milk!) leeches the body of its calcium reserves.

ENZYME SUPPLEMENTS

There has been some hype and misinformation spread in the raw-food movement on the topic of enzymes. I personally don't think that the raw diet gives results because of its enzyme-richness. I think it's more because the diet excludes foods that are not specific to human beings (grains, beans, meat, dairy, etc.), leaving only fruits, vegetables, nuts and seeds. In my opinion, cooking is not bad just because it destroys the enzymes, but mainly because it destroys vitamins and minerals and transforms complex substances like fats and protein into powerful toxins.

Here's an example of the hype: we are told to eat papayas because of enzymes. There are plenty of enzymes in green, unripe papayas. But as the fruit ripens, the enzymes convert all that starch into simple sugar. When the fruit is fully ripe, the enzymes are almost all gone! Strange? No, the enzymes are only needed by the fruit to transform complex substances (starch) into simple substances (sugar). They are not needed for digestion because the ripe fruit is fully digestible, without a lot of enzymes, if any at all.

Raw-foodists believe they spare their enzyme "reserves" by eating all-raw. But many foods contained in a typical raw diet not only contain few enzymes, but also use up the body's own digestive enzymes! For example: dried nuts and seeds, all oils (even cold-pressed), tahini and nut butters. Even sprouting does not entirely destroy the enzyme-inhibitors contained in beans and grains. They may contain a lot of enzymes, but they are difficult to digest due to the presence of these enzyme inhibitors (toxins that prevent the seed from sprouting) and raw starch.

There are many raw-foodists who take enzyme supplements. According to them, the foods we consume, even if they are raw, do not contain enough enzymes because they are picked mostly unripe and are sold weeks or months later. They are not fresh. Furthermore, modern humans, because of wrong living and eating habits, do not produce enough powerful digestive enzymes anymore.

So what should we think of enzyme supplements on a raw food diet? Are they needed or are they just another fad? I think that instead of worrying about enzymes, it is better to pay attention to your digestion first. If you don't feel or hear your organs; have no digestive pains and almost no gas, if your elimination is good, without bad odors or need for toilet paper, then your digestion — the purpose of dietary enzymes, anyway — is fine. Then why worry about enzymes? The enzymes in foods will not digest them for you. You can eat an enzyme-rich, wrongly combined meal and digest it poorly. The results will be fermentation (leading to lots of gas) and drained energy.

VITAMIN B12

Vitamin B12 is essential for health and it is not usually found in a strict vegan diet. Symptoms of B12 deficiency can include numbness in the hands and feet; unsteadiness and poor muscular coordination; and even cognitive deficits such as confusion, mental slowness and memory problems.

Normally, vitamin B12 is made in the intestinal flora of the intestines with the help of beneficial bacteria. If the intestinal flora is in good shape and if we eat some unwashed homegrown or wild greens, we should not suffer with this deficiency.

The most important thing is to make sure you do not destroy your intestinal flora with (in order of importance):

1. The use of antibiotics
2. Many prescribed drugs
3. Many popular herbal remedies that contain caffeine and multiple toxic substances
4. Herbal intestinal cleanses
5. Repeated colonics
6. Overeating, which causes food to ferment and produce an array of poisons and acids that will impair the intestinal flora.
7. Coffee, tea and other stimulants
8. An excess of acid fruits (for most people, more than 4-5 oranges, or 1-3 grapefruits a day)
9. Raw garlic, onions and strong, spicy foods and condiments, especially foods rich in mustard oil

If you believe that you may have partly destroyed your intestinal flora (the use of antibiotics is the main culprit), you may have reasons to worry about a vitamin B12 deficiency. In his article, *Vitamin B12 Recommendations for Total-Vegetarians*, Dr. Alan Goldhamer comments:

> Upon reflection, we should note that in a more primitive setting, human beings almost certainly would have obtained an abun-

dance of vitamin B12 from the bacterial "contamination" of unwashed fresh fruits and vegetables, regardless of their intake of animal products. Human vitamin B12 deficiency is very unlikely to occur in such a setting. Only very small amounts of dietary vitamin B12 are needed because our bodies do a fabulous job of recycling this essential nutrient. A person living in the ancestral environment regularly would have consumed fresh fruits and vegetables that were not consistently, fastidiously cleaned, as we routinely do today. Our current unusual degree of hygiene is useful for combating many health threats — but may leave long-term, strict vegans vulnerable to the potential problem of vitamin B12 deficiency.

So those eating homegrown or wild, unwashed plants will benefit from the useful bacteria found in these uncultivated vegetables.

Dr. Goldhamer continues, "Although most people associate vitamin B12 deficiency with vegan diets, the majority of cases occur among people who regularly consume animal products." I have heard the same thing from several doctors and naturopaths who have had experience with B12-deficient individuals. They are mostly meat eaters. It proves that a lack of B12 in the diet is not the main cause of this deficiency, since animal products contain this vitamin. A lack of absorption coupled with a destroyed intestinal flora are the culprits.

The most important things to do to avoid B12 deficiency, in order of importance are:

1.   Avoid everything that destroys intestinal flora.
2.   Include bacteria-rich, unwashed homegrown or wild greens in your diet.

To close, I will share a few thoughts that come to mind when I think about supplements, in no particular order:

•   My experience with many of these products is that they are an absolute waste of money.
•   If soil is depleted and the food grown in it is deficient, then so is the food used by supplement manufacturers.
•   These super-foods may contain tons of minerals per gram, but it would still take cups of the stuff to really make a difference.

Simply look at the labels and do the math.
•   The effects people get from supplements is often a drug effect. For example, dandelion greens contain a toxic substance, that we can easily detect by its bitter taste. That means that you could eat a few leaves but not much more. Your body will let you know when you've eaten too many. But if you juice it and force yourself to drink it down, you may feel a "buzz," which is nothing more than a toxic overload — in essence, a drugging effect. The same goes for hot peppers. If you eat several fresh hot peppers, you may feel a "buzz" due to the toxic substance capsaicin, contained in them.
•   Supplements are an easy way to feel better about your diet without changing anything.

I believe that supplementation is not necessary. Some fanatical supplement users may present arguments that may seem hard to refute, but their claims are rarely based on solid facts.

I think it is better to spend your money on whole, organic food rather than on supplements whose benefits are largely unproven.

11

HUNGER

When an individual has learned to live instinctively in every particular and eats only when genuinely hungry instead of for pleasure or out of fear of offending a host or hostess, then he or she is on the road to a state of superior health unmatched in modern times.

Virginia Vetrano, MD

Hunger is a lost mechanism, a forgotten sensation if you will. Most people eat without hunger, don't know what hunger is, and find learning to eat when truly hungry difficult. It may be the most difficult part of natural eating — learning to listen to our bodies again.

I could go on, but I wish to turn this section over to a classic text by Albert Mosséri. Only a few hygienists talk about hunger. You rarely hear anyone else talk about it anywhere else. *But this principle, one of the most difficult to follow because of our ill conditioning and bad eating habits, is of prime importance.*

THE PLEASURES OF HUNGER

"Popular and medical opinion holds hunger to be a painful and unbearable sensation. We hear about the pangs of hunger. 'I suffered from hunger,' some people will say to you! But hunger is a manifestation of the normal functioning of the body and all normal functions of the body bring pleasure. Urination, defecation, sight, sleep, sex: these are all pleasurable functions.

"Why, then, talk about the sufferings of hunger — its pains? It is true that certain individuals experience some pains — but these are signs of *elimination* and detoxification erasing the irritating consequences of previous meals. The person who stops smoking or drinking coffee experiences similar sufferings and similar pains coming from detoxification. These inconveniences should not lead to eating, smoking or drinking coffee.

"Let me reiterate: the sufferings felt are not those of hunger but those of *detoxification*. These sufferings disappear when detoxification is over. When hunger finally arrives, no suffering is felt.

TRUE AND FALSE HUNGER

"Every time I discuss the subject of hunger during my daily talks for those who come to fast at my house, some people say that they are hungry in the morning. This is why I wish to make the distinction between true and false hunger.

"False hunger disappears quickly, reappears again and disappears another time. On the other hand, true hunger persists and becomes stronger. So to distinguish them, we only have to wait for one hour, or even more. At the beginning hunger will be weak, but the more we wait, the more true hunger will be accentuated.

"In cases of malnutrition, acute hunger can lead to a sensation of fainting, passing out or collapsing. No work or anything else can be done before being fed. At this moment, one or two pieces of fruit should be eaten immediately, without any beverage.

" 'Appetite,' writes Shelton, 'is a counterfeit hunger, a creature of habit and cultivation and may be due to any one of a number of things; such as the arrival of the habitual meal time; the sight, taste, or smell of food; condiments and seasoning; or even the thought of food.'

"But this is not true hunger. Appetite is a false hunger.

"True hunger is not accompanied by any symptoms. There are no headaches, or any discomforts. Ideas are clear, the mind lucid; we are optimistic, happy, tranquil, serene. True hunger can manifest itself spontaneously at any time of the day but not during the night. During the night, the muscles, including the stomach, relax. The stomach is not ready to handle food during the night rest. However, if we feel true hunger before midnight, then a few leaves of lettuce should calm it and insure a good night sleep.

CHAPTER 11 — HUNGER

"Fletcher said that, in true hunger, 'water runs in the mouth.' But according to me, we need to wait one hour. True hunger persists, whereas false hunger, with all its morbid and deceptive symptoms, disappears.

CONTRACTED OR DISTENDED THROAT?

"Most professional Hygienists attribute the main role in the manifestation of hunger to the glands of the throat and the mouth. Shelton attributes this active, main role to the nerves. In fact, the nerves are really what command this sensation of emptiness and dilation in the esophagus and the throat.

"It is why during moments of fatigue, worry, anger and other negative feelings, even if food is needed, the body will not signal for it or manifest hunger. The nerves will keep the throat and esophagus contracted. When conditions are again favorable, hunger manifests itself in the dilation of the throat and esophagus.

A PLEASANT SENSATION

"True hunger is always a pleasant sensation, even if it is urgent. A hole in the stomach, an emptiness accompanied by rhythmical contractions, a sensation of relaxation that climbs from the stomach to the throat spanning the esophagus — all these symptoms are pleasant. On the other hand, in cases of malnutrition and lack of reserves, the person can experience a diffuse hunger, an incapacity to work and to concentrate. He feels faint. These sensations disappear quickly within a few weeks, as the reserves are filled up. The person will then feel hunger, but his mind will be alert, vivid and lucid and his mood, optimistic and serene.

FALSE HUNGER: LIKE A DRUG

"All the morbid symptoms of false hunger that I describe strikingly resemble the symptoms of withdrawal manifested in the smoker, the tea or coffee drinker and the drug addict when they stop taking their poison. These withdrawal symptoms are those of false hunger — they are elimination symptoms.

"False hunger is a symptom of elimination of the residues of previous meals. These symptoms are well-known by drug addicts, smokers, coffee and tea drinkers. Unfortunately, eaters ignore them. Addiction can exist both for drugs and unhealthy foods.

"It is obvious that if, during detoxification, a drug addict or a smoker takes his poison again, the unpleasant detoxification symptoms stops. But we should never stop detoxification, whether it stems from drug, alcohol, coffee, or unhealthy foods. 'The morbid symptoms of false hunger,' writes Shelton, 'are identical to those felt by drug users when they are deprived of their habitual drug.'

"Of course, the symptoms of addiction to drugs are much stronger, but addiction to food and the habit of fixed meal times end up in food intoxication and gluttony. They produce their own symptoms that we mistake for hunger.

"It is true that these symptoms are temporarily relieved by food intake, just like coffee temporarily relieves the headache caused by the previous cup of coffee! This is why we imagine and convince ourselves that we need to eat food. In the extreme case, the ulcer sufferers and those with a sick stomach eat often to relieve their stomach pains, but ultimately worsen their condition. It's a vicious circle they can only break with fasting. Otherwise, they go further down. All these morbid symptoms end up disappearing if we stop eating for a while and wait for true hunger.

"In his book *Perfect Health*, Haskell said that he, '...had asked thousands of people, including doctors, to describe the sensation of natural hunger. In their response, he noted the following symptoms: fainting, sensation of emptiness in the stomach, pains, etc. But all these sensation are those of appetite and not of hunger. They come from an incorrect way of eating.'

APPETITE AND HUNGER

"Shelton compares the appetite to the desire for nicotine, alcohol, coffee, tea, and chocolate. 'No one could ever be hungry for these poisonous substances," he writes. "In fact, they serve no physiological need and are thus always harmful. No physiological demand for these substances can ever occur.'

"It happens sometimes that appetite is accompanied by various sensations of discomforts, sensations of weakness, depression, stomach gnawings, rumblings in the stomach, nausea, headaches and other morbid sensations. Shelton, again: 'According to Dr. Claunch, true hunger can be distinguished from appetite in the following manner: 'When you are hungry and you feel well, it is true hunger.

But when you are apparently hungry and you feel unwell, it is false hunger.'

"I will however make an exception to this rule when the person feels faint. At the beginning of dietary change, digestion is weak, the cells are screaming for nourishment, and hunger becomes frequent and imperative.

"Some people can feel faint and should eat quickly at these moments. After that, with the improvement of the digestive power, the reserves will be more substantial — hunger will be felt less often and will be easier to bear. With the old diet of denatured and cooked foods, one digests only 20% and the rest exits in the stools the next day. However, with the new, healthy diet, composed of living foods, one digests 90% and the stools are in small quantities, well-formed and odorless. So the change from one state to another creates an urgent call for food, until the digestive power improves. This hunger is a symptom of undernourishment.

"However, in some people, a change of diet initiates an intense elimination and hunger disappears. Then it would be useful to start with a fast, as preparation for this new healthy diet. Dr. Claunch makes another useful distinction, 'When a sick person skips a habitual meal, he gets weak before feeling hunger. But when a healthy person skips a habitual meal, he feels hunger before getting weak.'

"Hunger is a sacred principle in our lives — a principle to respect at all times. Those who tell you to smell the foods to make your choice ignore hunger and are seeking appetite! The most common and worst mistake is to fill up our stomach because it's meal time, or because the doctor told us to, or as a social distraction to please our host and guests.

A NATURAL DEMAND

"When we eat without experiencing a natural demand, we don't benefit, or we benefit very little, from what we eat. It is exactly like those who practice deep and forced breathing without any need, or those who drink without being thirsty. 'This way of eating,' writes Shelton, 'transforms the body into a fertilizer factory.'

"True hunger represents a natural demand, and furthermore, it indicates that food will be effectively assimilated by the body. On the other hand, when we smell foods before choosing a tempting one, we are looking to increase appetite. We only digest a part of what we ingest.

WHAT HUNGER IS NOT

" 'To understand what true hunger is,' writes Shelton, 'let's see what it is not, before trying to find what it is. Think about thirst: is it a pain? A feeling of dizziness? Of passing out? None of this. Thirst is felt in the mouth and in the throat and we feel a conscious desire to drink water. We never mistake a headache for thirst, because we know thirst very well. It is the same for genuine hunger. We feel a genuine desire to eat, we are at ease, without pains or discomforts. The saliva runs abundantly in the mouth and often we desire a particular food.'

"Some fasting patients feel acute stomach pains that may last for a week. It is not hunger. Those that feel this are dyspeptics, nervous and anxious individuals, ulcer sufferers and those that suffer from gastritis because of unhealthy foods and medicines.

"Certain temporary pains are due to the spasmodic contractions of the stomach and intestines, coming from the psychological or emotional disturbance of the sympathetic, abdominal nerve that controls this region of the body.

SYMPTOMS OF TRUE HUNGER	SYMPTOMS OF FALSE HUNGER
• The stomach "aspirates" • The mouth salivates • The mind is optimistic, clear, and happy • A pleasant sensation in the throat • Hunger persists when we wait	• Dry mouth, coated tongue, bad breath • Headaches • Rumblings in the stomach • The mind is spacy, unclear, the spirit pesimistic • Stomach cramps and pains, nausea • Hunger disappears when we wait

WHEN WE FEEL FAINT

"According to Dr. Doods, the sensation of fainting, in certain cases, does not come from a lack of food, but rather from the absence of a habitual stimulant. But this could be objected to. In fact, this sensation should not be ignored or taken lightly. The subjects suffer from severe undernourishment because they digest only 10% of what they eat. We cannot prolong this state without risk. These persons must be fed appropriately, in small quantities at a time, with repeated small meals, in favorable conditions of rest (before and after every meal) and in the absence of all disturbance, psychological, emotional or otherwise. Shelton also mentions the sensation of fainting among the sensations of false hunger, but I consider this to be an acute symptom of undernourishment and genuine hunger.

"Let's examine more closely this sensation of fainting, an issue of gravity. When this happens, the person should eat, because the body is signaling for food and lie down a little while. After some weeks, this type of hunger disappears, to be replaced by an nonurgent hunger, when the reserves are restored.

"Thus, those that feel this fainting sensation for having missed a single meal should be fed in this manner. I have encountered many similar cases of people who have consciously ignored this sensation of hunger. They kept on not eating and ended up with an uncontrollable bulimia that resulted in death by undernourishment. In this state, large meals are not properly digested. They pass in the stools and exacerbate this state of undernourishment. They can lead to death by inanition. What is required in these extreme conditions is many small meals, under the control of an energetic supervisor who will not let the person gorge himself to death, but will allow him to eat just enough to calm his hunger.

WHEN WE FEEL WEAK

"We must not mistake this faint sensation for weakness. In this case, we feel no strength, incapable of concentrating or making any physical effort. This is due to toxemia. The overloaded liver takes up all the blood and energy, which deprives the muscles. In these moments, one should abstain from eating, lie down and postpone the meal. The strength will come back quickly, along with mental clarity.

"However when a person feels faint — an emptiness inside, a state close to passing out, a diffuse hunger that goes from the stomach and climbs up to the throat and mouth — the person should eat a little bit and then rest or take a nap. These persons can carry a few dates with them, just in case.

"Weakness, on the other hand, is not a symptom of hunger, but one of poisoning. It calls not for a cup of coffee, a cigarette or food — as is the habit of most people — but a rest, *lying down*. Some people will object that in normal life, we don't always have the occasion to lie down when we are tired and that a cigarette or a cup of coffee "wakes you up" and enables you to pursue your activities. I always reply that this happens to the detriment of one's health and that, sooner or later, one will suffer the consequences. There is always a bill to pay.

THE SMELL OF FOODS AND CONDIMENTS
"Contrary to what is practiced by the instinctos (those who follow instinctotherapy), true hunger cannot be aroused by the smell, taste, or even the thought of a food. These instinctos, who sniff foods before eating them, are not hungry, but are only looking for appetite and desire. When we are truly hungry, we are not so picky in our food choices.

"On the other hand, true hunger is not stimulated by condiments, spices and salt. These substances are poisons. The saliva that pours over salt does not contain digestive juices, but water to dilute the poison and render it less corrosive to the tissues.

"When we feel true hunger, we are satisfied by simple food of any type in the natural state — without any seasoning or preparation. When we feel true hunger, we generally don't have a preference for a particular food that our sense of smell is instinctively supposed to locate and pick out. *Hunger is the best sauce.*

"However, in false hunger, one is looking for desire and appetite. One is difficult and picky and as to smell foods one after the other, to choose only one food at the end. This is the 'instincto' practice.

VARIETY EXCITES APPETITE
"It is known that appetite, desire and false hunger can be stimulated by variety. When we no longer want to eat a food we are full

of, we can excite the appetite by changing to another food. This is why variety leads to gluttony.

"Do we have to limit ourselves to only one kind of food per meal? Maybe. Anyway, we should not multiply the number of foods — two to three types of fruit are better than five or six. 'How many people are still hungry when it is time for dessert?' asks Shelton. 'But even so, very few refuse this dessert!'

HOW MANY MEALS A DAY?

"I often get asked: how many meals we should eat each day. One, two, three? It depends on your hunger. There is no sacred number. If you eat small meals, like vegetarian animals, you will need to eat three, four or even five meals a day. But if you eat large meals, like the carnivores, then one or two meals will suffice.

SIMPLE FOODS

"In my opinion, any food can satisfy true hunger. On the other hand, in false hunger the person is only satisfied in the capricious choice of a particular food, according to his smell or his taste. This is why the practice of smelling foods one at a time before making a choice reflects false hunger."

Notes By F.P. — When you think that you are hungry, it is good to wait an hour before eating. If it is true hunger, your pleasure when eating will be even greater and you will not be able to ingest large quantities of foods, because the stomach will not be distended by previous meals.

When you are truly hungry, any food can satisfy you, but sometimes we desire one category of food in particular — fruit or vegetables. When you are truly hungry, a simple apple or a head of lettuce will seem like a delight of the gods. It is through hunger that eating simple, unseasoned foods becomes natural and easy.

To start the practice of eating only when hungry, begin with the morning meal. Hunger rarely occurs in the first two hours after waking up. In most people, it takes at least 3-4 hours and sometimes more. To avoid being impatient, drink some water, converse, take a walk, rest, read, work or exercise. Avoid cleaning your mouth in the morning because a coated tongue and bad breath are signs of elimination, a no-no to eating. When you are hungry, your mouth will naturally clear up in the morning and salivate abundantly.

If you eat before going to sleep, you are not likely to sleep well, because the digestion of food will interfere with sleep. If that happens, the next day true hunger may not manifest itself before 3-4 p.m. So avoid eating or drinking three hours before going to bed.

12

SLEEP

The mode of living in this age produces such a waste of power and such a sense of weariness that only the limited few ever know the supreme delights and the enviable luxury of power in reserve. They keep up their semblance of vigor by means of stimulation and seldom take sufficient time to re-charge their vital or nervous batteries. Nights are turned into day, while mental and nervous poise is exceedingly rare. All poison habits, all excesses, the indulgence of any or all the passions constitute distinct drains upon the vital resources and are sources of diminished vitality, crippled usefulness and shortened life. Modern life presents us with an almost unlimited variety of means of stimulation, excitement, thrills and dissipation chiefly originating in the clever but perverted ingenuity of those who reap financial rewards from these things.

Herbert Shelton
Orthobionomics

SLEEP AND DIET

You may have heard that raw-foodists only need to sleep 5-6 hours per day. I met some people who told me they only needed 3-4 hours of sleep a day. I even met one man who said he slept 2 hours a day. Impressed by this, I tried everything to be able to sleep less: juice fasting, fruit diets, etc. But I still needed my 7-9 hours of sleep.

Although it is true that the need for sleep is affected by diet, the amount of sleep required may not be the same from one person to another. In fact, the only good advice I can give you is to sleep as much as you want! And if you are trying to overcome a health challenge, the more the better!

An observation of nature will show us that animals love to rest and sleep. They get as much sleep as they wish, which, of course, depends on the species. Also, we notice that young animals need more sleep than mature ones. The same holds true for humans. The younger you are, the more you need to sleep. And it is good for the elderly to get plenty of sleep. (Surveys show that elderly do not get the amount of sleep they truly need.)

THE IMPORTANCE OF SLEEP

Sleep and rest are essential to recharge our nervous energy. Our physical, emotional and mental balance depends on the quality and the quantity of our sleep. Work and play is great, but it also puts a demand on the body, dissipates our energy, and fills our tissues with toxins. Rest is the only thing that recharges these "batteries" and allows for the proper elimination of metabolic wastes (toxins).

It may be true that the healthier we are, the less rest and sleep we need. But since we live in such a rotten and polluted modern world, we probably would be better off securing even more rest. And all those with health challenges must get the maximum amount rest, while at the same time avoiding mental and physical exertion if they are to heal.

> "If invalids are to be restored to good health, if strength and vigor are to take the place of debility and weakness, we must save life, by saving power. The conditions of recovery are conditions of conservation and recuperation. This principle applies to every organ and function of the body. Rest for each organ is as imperative as rest for the whole body. The heart requires rest as much as do the muscles and the arms. The stomach must have rest the same as the eyes. The glands of the body have the same need for rest as does the brain. Rest, by reducing activity, is the first requisite of recovery."
>
> Herbert Shelton
> *Orthobionomics*

A bad piece of advice commonly given to chronically sick people is to get more exercise. However, the further depletion of energy caused by exercising when they should be resting, makes their recovery difficult. There is no danger in stopping all physical exercise and getting as much rest as possible for a few months. It is also my advice to those changing to a raw diet to get as much rest and sleep as possible, to temporarily suspend all hard, physical work, and to let your body heal. After a few months, the weight will start to come back and then you can exercise again to build up strength.

ADVICE FOR BETTER SLEEP

Try to sleep at regular hours. Wake up early and don't go to bed late at night. You have heard this before! In a world of roisterers and party-junkies, going to bed early and at regular hours may sound boring. However, if you choose to be healthy, that's what needs to be done. It is not part of our natural cycle to go to bed at 3 a.m. and wake up at noon. It is not part of our natural cycle to go to bed one day at 9 p.m. and the next at 1 am. We are affected by this more than you can imagine. Paul Nison says, "The most common mistakes raw-foodists make are eating too much and not sleeping enough." I would add sleeping at irregular hours and going to bed late at night. A old saying is, "The hours before midnight count for double." We may well have invented electric bulbs, but night is still meant for sleeping and daytime for waking.

If you have trouble sleeping, it may be caused by several things. Anything containing caffeine, especially if you eat a raw diet, will disturb your sleep. A few years ago I drank herbal teas and green tea daily. I read somewhere that the caffeine content in green tea was negligible. I couldn't fall asleep before 3 a.m. and it took me months to make the connection.

Other foods that disturb sleep are: garlic, spices, onions, condiments and the habit of eating late at night. Your evening meal should be fairly simple, light and properly combined. Also, avoid eating sweet fruit in the evening. The sugar and acids in fruit may prevent you from falling asleep, and they may also disturb your sleep. I recommend not eating or drinking three hours before going to sleep. Otherwise, your sleep will be disturbed by digestion, which will manifest as disturbing dreams and nightmares. What we eat before going to sleep greatly influences how we feel the next day.

If you are hungry before midnight, a few bites of raw vegetables, such as lettuce or bell pepper, should be enough. But avoid fruits and fats. Otherwise, you may wake up tired the next day.

13

WATER

OUR WATER NEEDS

On a diet of raw fruits and vegetables, without salt, spices, condiments and without too many nuts or avocados, one needs to drink little water. This is because juicy fruits and vegetables contain all or most of the water the body needs. The recommendation of drinking eight glasses of water a day is for those eating a seed-based, mostly cooked diet (bread, meat, cheese and starches) that is low in water and high in salt, fat and protein.

Raw-foodists who are not training athletes and feel they need to drink lots of water are probably eating salt, spices and condiments, as well as too many nuts and seeds or too many avocados. If you don't make these mistakes, you won't normally feel the need to drink much water, except when the body really needs it, such as in times of warm weather and during intense exercise. However, during detoxification crises — headaches, stomach pains, etc. — we should drink a lot water to help flush out the toxins.

Gorillas and the other great apes drink almost no water. Sometimes they'll slurp the water accumulated inside a fluted leaf, which doesn't account for much considering the size of these beasts. Their water needs are met by the water-rich fruits and vegetables they eat.

The best waters to use are distilled, reverse-osmosis, or filtered water. In America, I would avoid drinking tap water everywhere, but in some other countries it is acceptable.

DRINKING TOO MUCH

Drinking too much water on a water-rich diet may dilute the content of the intestines, which, by osmotic pressure will cause poisons to be absorbed — leading to headaches and other discomforts. Drinking a few glasses of water during the day is good, but if you stick to fruits and vegetables and you avoid salt and condiments, you probably won't need to drink more than that in a day.

UNNATURAL THIRST

You may feel *unnatural thirst* if you make a mistake in eating: food that is poorly combined, overeating nuts, seeds or avocados; overeating dried fruit; or eating something with salt or cheese. You can thus monitor your digestion with the thirst factor. If you feel unnatural thirst often it means you are making mistakes.

You may also feel *unnatural thirst* if you overeat sweet fruit. Eating too much sugar will cause the body to reject the excess in urine with water — leading to a dry mouth.

Unnatural thirst is an unpleasant sensation. It is one of dryness in the mouth and may be accompanied by slight dizziness. Natural thirst, in contrast, is a pleasant sensation, like natural hunger. It manifests itself as a strong, slightly exciting desire for water.

WHEN TO DRINK

Water is important during transition. The body dilutes toxins and carries them out with it. Drink as much as a liter upon rising from sleep and enough throughout the day to prevent a dry mouth. Later you will find that your need and desire for additional water will decrease.

A friend of mine has found water extremely effective in instantly banishing cravings. He says the cravings seem to be calls from the body for help, in the form of water, to eject residues of the very food he is craving. Just one or two swallows, at any time of day, does it.

There are times when drinking a water is crucial. One is during a fast, when no other food is taken. Also, when experiencing a detoxification crisis, it is good to drink an adequate amount of water to help rush the toxins out. If you exercise a lot, you need to drink additional water even on a fruit and vegetable diet — as much as a gallon a day, according to Dr. Doug Graham, trainer of world champion athletes. You will eventually get to know exactly how much water you need to perform at your best.

14

RAW RECIPES

COMBO-ABOMBOS

RC Dini, author of the infamous classic "Raw Courage World," coined the term "combo-abombo." A combo-abombo is a combination that is an abomination. In other words, a poorly combined recipe.

The raw-food cuisine is supposed to be the healthiest cuisine ever, because only raw and living ingredients are used. Juliano, the famous raw chef, says in his book, "I believe eating Raw is the healthiest and most harmonious way for us and the planet. However, I am offering you a wealth of suggestions so you can balance whatever lifestyle you choose with delicious, superior, gourmet food that enriches your body, mind and soul." (Raw: The Uncook Book, page VII)

To avoid the pitfall of cooked food, raw-foodists have created an array of raw recipes that resemble their favorite cooked dishes. Let's take a look at a popular raw food recipe called the "Nut Loaf," which is supposed to imitate a meat loaf and which contains, among other things:

- 1 1/3 cups cashews
- 1 1/3 cups sunflower seeds
- 1 1/3 cups almonds
- 1/2 cup oil

This serves two. Let's take a closer look. The fat content of the nuts and oil used in the recipe is as follows:

- cashews: 1 1/3 cups = 150 grams = 69.5 grams fat
- sunflower seeds: 1 1/3 cups = 190 grams = 94.2 grams fat
- almonds: 1 1/3 cups = 200 grams = 104.4 g fat
- olive oil: 1/2 cup = 125 grams = 125 grams fat.

TOTAL: 393.1 grams fat
For each person: 196.55 grams fat!

So each person consumes almost an entire cup of oil in this recipe! And I have seen people eat more! But what would be the consequences of sitting down and drinking a cup of oil?

I looked at an extreme example, just too show you how crazy raw-food recipes can get. I will say that most raw-foodists have enough common sense to avoid these recipes most of the time, but often they don't realize that these combinations are a slippery slope — a steep one — and lead to sheer abuse.

The use of salt, spices, soy sauce, miso, onion, garlic and oil excites the palate and leads to overeating. This is not food that will give you health and energy. It reminds me of all the products vegetarians have created to replace meat: tofu hot-dogs, gardenburgers and the like. But a vegetarian doesn't want anything that resembles meat. She is over her meat addiction and is not seeking to replace it with foods that resemble it. Oftentimes, these foods are not healthy. In fact, they only slightly healthier than the real thing. Likewise, a raw-foodist doesn't strive to create foods that resemble the popular meals she ate in the past.

The ideal is to limit recipes to combinations with a few ingredients that are properly combined. Dr. Doug Graham has a rule that I like. He calls it the 5-5-5 rule. It means that you should eat meals that take less than 5 minutes to prepare, with a maximum of 5 ingredients, and that cost less than $5.

SOCIAL EATING

As raw-foodists, we may not be ready to give up the social aspects of eating. Some may view our sitting down to munch on lettuce and avocados with our bare hands as uncultured, as if we were "eating like animals." They will prefer to prepare recipes and serve everyone his meal on a fancy plate. But you don't have to give up good table manners when eating "rabbit food." We can still present simple foods artistically on the plate in a way that appeals to the eye as well as to the palate.

Once in a while, you will find yourself invited by other raw-foodists for a meal of fancy recipes. Or maybe you'll want to try that new raw restaurant. So you'll be tempted to eat a few combo-abombos. Okay, fine. Enjoy it. It is not healthy to be fanatical or repressive. But we also have to think in advance and recognize the food for what it is, and how it is going to make us feel afterwards, especially if we eat a lot of it. By now we are well aware that just because some food may be raw, that doesn't automatically make it healthy.

In Montreal, we organize potlucks once a month. The last time, we made a "sac du marché" potluck, which means "produce bag potluck." It involves going to the market (or garden), selecting one or two kinds of fruits and vegetables, and bringing them in the bag. We then wash everything at the potluck and maybe cut and arrange the fruits and vegetables artistically on a plate. But no mixing! It's a hit.

Complicated raw recipes are "gateway foods" to worse things. They are gateways to junk food, overeating, indigestion and confusion.

15

SALT, SPICES AND CONDIMENTS

Pure food can make a poet of you:

> There is nothing that entices us with greater appeal, nothing that awakens the desire to eat, nothing that arouses every organ of digestion and pleases the sense of taste more than Nature's richly colored, delicately flavored, highly scented, luscious and odorous edibles.
>
> He who is accustomed to eating unseasoned, unspiced foods knows that condiment users are missing many fine, delicate flavors that are far more pleasing to the sense of taste than any sauce, relish, or spice can ever be. Real pleasure in eating comes from tasting the natural flavors in foods.
>
> *Herbert Shelton*

Nature offers us simple foods that taste good without salt, seasonings, condiments, herbs, spices and other flavorings. Unfortunately, most of us have been raised on highly seasoned and salted foods, so we have difficulty returning to a simple, plain diet. We may even view such a diet as spartan or ascetic. Rawfoodists may refrain from using ketchup, mustard and the like, but many of them use dried spices, aromatic herbs and sometimes even salt. I included them in my recipe book "The Sunfood Cuisine," though I stated that it was possible to make the recipes delicious without salt and spices.

I recommend we avoid these substances. They are slightly toxic and very irritating to a purified body. Even though I always knew that these condiments were not the best, it took me a while to realize their true nature. I thought their consequences were negligible. I was wrong!

At some point I realized that even aromatic herbs and mild spices like curry had to be avoided. I was feeling itchy all the time for no apparent reason. When I discontinued the herbs and spices, the itchiness went away. The effects are not obvious to most people, but they are to those who have been living on a more natural diet. Salt may also cause itching in a purer body.

That being said, it doesn't mean that you have to fanatically refuse to taste something because it has some cumin powder in it. It is best to avoid salt and spices without making a religion out of it.

SALT

The body needs sodium, but in small quantities. We get it from the fruits and vegetables we eat. Good tomatoes taste a little salty. Celery, spinach and dark greens are naturally salty. Some apples are too. That's sodium. But sodium chloride, the most popular condiment in the world, is an inorganic mineral compound that the body has no use for. Table salt is not metabolized by the body the way organic sodium is. It is a poison that the body must reject with effort.

Salt kills life, which is why we preserve foods in salt — it prevents living activity from occurring. It is an antibiotic, which means "anti-life." If you put salt on a fresh cut in your skin, you will be able to feel its effects for yourself. It will burn you.

Salt is not broken down or used by the body and must be rejected. But since the average person consumes so much salt in one day, this task is never fully accomplished. So the salt accumulates in the body. It causes the body to retain water in order to dilute the salt in the tissues, and to prevent harming the cells. Excess salt is deposited at various places in the body, such as on the walls of the arteries. Blood flow is thereby disrupted, and high blood pressure is the result.

Sea salt is not much better than other types of salt. Sea salt is just rock salt diluted by the ocean. The body has no use for it.

Whenever you eat sea salt you are eating a type of inorganic salt that your body does not use and has to reject.

Before the Europeans arrived on this continent, native peoples did not use salt and were in excellent health. Many cultures throughout the world never used salt until this poison was introduced to them by the Europeans. After its inclusion into their diet, their health progressively deteriorated, although there were several contributing factors to this deterioration.

Animals don't eat salt unless they get tempted into licking a salt source somewhere in nature, which rarely happens. Their instinct is better than ours but not 100% perfect. They can also make mistakes and be fooled by salt. Anyhow, salt licks are rare and most animals never have access to them.

When you stop eating salt, it will take many months for your body to reject it. Some days you may taste salt in your mouth, although you may not have eaten it in weeks. It is another proof that the body is rejecting the salt and not using it. You may urinate more at night for a while, even many months, until the body has rejected all the salt. Complete "desalinization" of the body may take years.

To replace salt, I have come up with a natural seasoning using celery. Simply dehydrate slices of celery (in very large quantities) in a dehydrator or oven (open, at low temperature). When they are completely dried, turn them into a powder using a coffee grinder. This will make a nice, naturally salty seasoning that you can use to replace salt. You can do the same with other vegetables to add additional flavor to this seasoning. Dried purple cabbage powder is especially good in salads.

SPICES
These include curry powder, cinnamon, black pepper, cloves, etc. They are made from roots, barks or leaves of different plants and they all taste bitter, hot, or otherwise unpleasant when eaten alone. They are all toxic to some degree. Nutmeg is even a powerful, hallucinogen when eaten in sufficient quantities.

AROMATIC HERBS
This category includes all herbs used for cooking: sage, thyme, basil, etc. These plants are too bitter or unpleasant to eat alone.

This is because they contain toxic elements. If you go a while without any herbs, spices and salt and eat them again, you will notice an unusual thirst and maybe even itchiness. I admit that their scent is fascinating and their flavor, when mixed with other foods, is pleasant. The occasional use of fresh parsley, basil, dill, or cilantro is okay. But I would avoid oregano, sage, rosemary, thyme and all herbs with a very strong taste.

RAW GARLIC, ONIONS, LEEKS

These fresh spices are used raw and cooked all over the world. They contain mustard oil which, unless oxidized by cooking or long exposure to air, is an irritant that greatly upsets the digestive tract. Some raw-foodists eat a lot of these foods and therefore carry a constant, unpleasant onion odor and breath.

I find that if I eat raw onions and garlic, I will get an unpleasant taste in my mouth hours later. If you like the taste, you can chop some onion or garlic and rinse them with warm water, or dehydrate them to evaporate some of the mustard oil. Also, when chopped in a food processor, onions lose a lot of their mustard oil through oxidation.

I also found a healthy condiment made with garlic flowers. It simply consists of garlic flowers chopped and mixed with sunflower oil. It has the wonderful garlic flavors but without the ill-effects. When the plant matures the mustard oil goes away. You can also use garlic greens. Simply plant garlic cloves in some soil (can be done indoors) and use the greens and flowers of the plant. Same with onions.

HOT PEPPERS

Hot peppers are especially toxic. They contain capsaicin, which is a very poisonous substance. You can easily prove to yourself the toxicity of hot peppers by observing your body's reactions after eating them. The mouth salivates and the nose often runs with clear mucus or water. These are ways for the body to dilute the poison. The warm feeling that we get is the irritation of the digestive tract and stomach. The body temperature often rises as the body tries to get rid of this strong, toxic substance.

Another argument against hot peppers and spices, is that children will refuse them. No one would give a hot pepper to a child.

Pregnant and nursing women are advised to avoid them. Apparently, the taste of garlic and onions and the spiciness of hot peppers can be tasted in milk the day after the mother eats them (though I have never had the chance to verify this). It would be another proof that the body is rejecting the toxins found in these foods. Mother's milk doesn't taste like strawberries after she eats them because these fruits are not toxic.

"But Frédéric," you say. "I can imagine living without salt, but don't you think you're going a bit far? How will I enjoy my food without seasonings and spices?"

Surprising things happen when you live on a salt-free, spice-free diet. You start to taste food again! The subtle, intense flavors of natural foods are imperceptible to the dulled palate of the condiment eater. After a while, you don't even miss them. If you happen to taste them again, you quickly perceive their toxicity. You have to try it yourself!

16

FOOD COMBINING

Shelton, the avenger:

> "The Earl of Sandwich is credited with having invented the sandwich — a modern dietetic abomination. The hamburger, a similar abomination, is also a modern dietetic innovation. Egg sandwiches, cheese sandwiches, ham sandwiches and similar protein-starch combinations are of recent origin. Dr. Tilden used to say that Nature never produced a sandwich. How true are his words!"
>
> *The Science and Fine Art of Food and Nutrition.*

SIMPLICITY IN EATING

We should be eating one food at a time and never mixing together anything. In the Garden of Eden, we satisfied our thirst and hunger under the mango tree and ate a few leaves from the plants growing under it. When we felt hunger again, we ate under the fig tree and so on. But going back to that simplicity is very difficult in our complicated world. So this is why we have to know how to properly combine our foods in order to avoid fermentation and putrefaction. When your digestion is fine, then everything else works better.

Quantities of food also matter. Two or three almonds probably combine with anything. When we eat more than two or three, they only combine well with certain foods. And any foods eaten in excess will lead to fermentation and putrefaction, whether they are combined well with other foods or not.

With a simple, mainly raw diet, we automatically avoid most bad food combining. In a traditional diet, everything is mixed together in every possible way. Ease of digestion is not the goal, but rather the excitement of the senses within one meal. When we are used to eating cooked, spicy, fatty, salted foods, it is difficult to appreciate the flavors of unadulterated fruits and vegetables. It took time to learn to eat this way, just like it took time for the smoker to learn to enjoy smoking and the alcoholic to learn to enjoy whiskey. It will take time to *unlearn* it, as well.

Whenever we combine foods in a dish or during a meal, it must be done in a way that these combinations digest easily. Bad food combining creates indigestion, fermentation and gas. All these signs, commonly considered normal, are indications of digestive malfunction — food is fermenting and putrefying in the intestines. Instead of feeding the body, the food poisons it. But we want that food to nourish, not poison us. So that's why it pays off to observe a few simple food combining rules.

I won't go into the whys and wherefores of these combinations. These simple rules are the result of scientific observation of human digestive physiology and the experience of thousands of people for two hundred years. If you wish to further explore this interesting topic, there are many excellent books available. I recommend a booklet by Dennis Nelson called *Food Combining Simplified* as well as *Food Combining Made Easy by* Dr. Herbert Shelton.

I will examine the combining of natural foods and only touch on the others.

FOOD CATEGORIES

Fruit

Acid: citrus, pineapple, lemon, tomato, berries, etc.
Sub-Acid: mild tree fruits: peach, apple, apricot, cherry, cherimoya, pear, etc.
Sweet: banana, papaya, fig, raisins, date, persimmons, many tropical, non-acidic fruits and dried fruit.
Melons: all kinds.

Vegetables

No/low starch: cucumber*, bell pepper*, dark greens (spinach, kale, etc.), cabbage, raw carrot and jicama.
Celery & lettuce
Starchy (cooked): potato, yam, carrot, steamed vegetables.

Fatty foods

Fruits: avocado, fresh olives.
Nuts and Seeds: walnuts, almonds, pecans, sunflower seeds, etc.
Oils and Fats: preserved olives, oils and butter.

*These foods are technically fruits but included in this category because of their composition.

SIMPLIFIED FOOD COMBINING

Combination propriety
Combine well = This combination is good with normal quantities of food.
May combine = This combination could be accepted by some people, but there are some reasons to avoid it for many.
Do not combine = This combination should be avoided.

Sweet fruits — *combine well* will with other varieties of sweet fruit, celery and lettuce. They *may combine* with acid fruit, melons, subacid fruit and non-starchy vegetables. They *do not combine* well with, starchy vegetables, avocado, nuts, seeds, oils and fats.

Acid Fruits — *combine well* with other varieties of acid fruits, sub acid fruits, celery and lettuce. They *may combine* with non-starchy vegetables and avocados. They *do not combine* well with starchy vegetables, nuts, seeds, oils and fats.

Melons — they only *combine well* with other varieties of melons.

Non-starchy vegetables — they *combine well* with all other vegetables, nuts, seeds, avocados, fats and oils. They *may combine* with fruit. They *do not combine* well with melons.

Lettuce and celery — they *combine well* with everything.

Starchy vegetables — they *combine well* with other vegetables. They *may combine* with avocado, oils and fats. They *do not combine* well with fruit, nuts and seeds.

Nuts and seeds — they *combine well* with non-starchy vegetables. They *combine very well* with tomatoes. They *do not combine* well with starchy vegetables, fruit, avocados, oils and fats.

Avocado — *combines well* with non-starchy vegetables (including celery and lettuce). It *may combine* with starchy vegetables, acid fruit, and oils. It *does not combine* well with nuts, seeds, sub-acid fruits and melons.

Oils and Fats — they *combine well* with non-starchy vegetables. They *may combine* with starchy vegetables. They *do not combine* well with fruit, nuts and seeds.

OTHER TRANSITION FOODS

Sprouted bread — combines with non-starchy vegetables and may combine with acid fruit.

Yogurt (soy or dairy) — combines with acid fruit, lettuce, celery and other non-starchy vegetables.

COMBINING INFERIOR FOODS

Meat & Fish — Eat in very small quantity, one kind only and combine with no/low starch vegetables only.

Bread — Eat as little as possible. Combines well with vegetables and fat.

Other Cereals — Eat as little as possible. Combine with vegetables only.

Junk Food — (Crackers and chips, candy, pastries, chocolate, etc.) These items do not combine with anything. If you happen to eat them, eat them away from the healthy meals so that digestion is neither hindered nor deranged.

17

DIGESTION

Instead of seeking the latest super-food or supplement or trying various therapies, pay attention to your digestion. When foods putrefy and ferment, they end up poisoning you. Poisons are reabsorbed in the intestines and may be the cause for headaches and many discomforts.

The quality of your digestion depends on many factors, such as the state of mind when eating, what foods are eaten, the degree of hunger, the strength of digestion, food combining, the quantities of food eaten, etc.

JUDGE YOUR DIGESTION

You can judge the quality of your digestion by taking a look at your stools. They should be:

- Quick
- Non-staining (no need for toilet paper)
- Without gas or bad odor

Bad-smelling stools, gas, noise in the stomach, pains — which are considered normal — are signs of indigestion. A dried mouth, when living mostly on fruits and vegetables, is also a sign of indigestion.

The quality of your sleep will also depend on digestion. If you eat too much or late at night, your sleep will be disturbed, sometimes by nightmares.

When you wake up in the morning, you should not have any burps, gas, noise in the stomach, or any sign that digestion is still going on in your stomach. If you do, then it means that digestion went on all night (depriving you of sleep) and is still going on in the morning. In order to correct the situation, fast until you feel true hunger and proceed to eat small amounts of properly combined food.

There are many causes for poor digestion:

• **Eating without hunger** — When the body needs no food and thus gives no signals for it, digestion is ineffective.
• **Poor-food combining** — Properly combining your meals will avoid many digestive problems. The mono-eater, who eats one food at a time, enjoys superior digestion.
• **Poor eating conditions** — Eating in a hurry or in a noisy or polluted atmosphere hinders digestion. Let us eat when we are relaxed and in a nice environment. Also, negative emotions like fear, worry and anxiety, instantly suspend the secretion of digestive juices. Under these conditions, it is imperative that we fast until we are relaxed and happy.
• **Overeating** — When overeaten, even the best foods will not digest properly. If you eat too much you end up digesting little of it.
• **Eating non-specific foods** — Many commonly consumed foods are not meant to be eaten by humans, and thus digest poorly even when properly combined. But when you stick to our specific foods (see chapter 22) you will be sure to enjoy excellent digestion.
• **Use of salt, spices, condiments** — These substances, as we have seen, are highly toxic. They will also impair and disturb digestion. Spiced foods are usually rejected, often causing diarrhea.

THE SNAKE METHOD

A snake can eat many eggs in a few hours. But it cannot eat eggs, lizards and birds, one right after the other. It knows that it needs eggs one day and not mice. The next time it eats, the snake will, perhaps, eat mice, but it never mixes them with other foods.

The practical application for us is obvious. We are told not to eat between meals to avoid disturbing digestion. Of course, when you eat two big meals a day, this rule makes sense. But when you eat small meals composed of one type of food only, the rule is not the same.

You can eat every two hours, as long as you are hungry and as long you eat the same food (like the snake), or at least the same kind of food. You can eat a couple apples every two hours. Or you can eat a bunch of grapes, then, two hours later, you can eat a couple apples. Two hours later you might eat a another bunch of grapes, etc. But we should avoid eating an apple and one hour later, a handful of nuts, and then two hours later, vegetables. If we want to change the type of foods we are eating, to switch from fruit to avocado as an example, using the snake method, we would wait until the digestion of one kind of food is complete — which can take a few hours. For example, say you eat two apples at noon. One hour later you'd like to eat an avocado. But you are still digesting the apple. They would conflict. Either wait to eat the avocado, or eat another apple or other sub-acid fruit.

ASSIMILATION

People worry that the foods they eat do not contain enough minerals. But even the best, organic foods, when poorly digested, bring little to the body. When your digestion works well, you can get all the vitamins and minerals you need from fruits and vegetables. When it works poorly, then it won't help to consume "superfoods." There are also other causes of poor assimilation. Digestion and assimilation are not the same. Assimilation is the cells' use of digested nutrients. This also can be faulty, as has been explained in *Just Eat An Apple*, #3 (Autumn, 2002).

18

JUICING AND BLENDING

IS IT NATURAL?

To eat a natural diet you don't need any appliances: neither blender, dehydrator, nor juicer. However, some of these machines can be useful and interesting for varying the diet. Beginners usually get a kick out of buying a juicer or a special blender, whereas more experienced raw-foodists tend to prefer keeping things simple. Personally, I sold my Green Power juicer one year ago and almost never miss it. But I still have a big, heavy-duty blender that I use quite a bit.

Blending is preferable to juicing, but some juices are good, too. There is nothing special about fruit and vegetable juices. They have no special healing power and they can even be considered inferior to whole foods. They are a food, but with the fiber removed. Yet fiber is important and was included by nature in fruits and vegetables for a reason. Removing the fiber creates a concentrated food that is assimilated too fast by the body. This is why I don't recommend juices often, and or in large quantities. Even though they may be a concentrated source of vitamins, the body rejects most of them. The body can never benefit from excesses.

HOW TO DRINK JUICES

This is not to say that juices are useless and can never be consumed. Vegetable juices in small quantities (8 oz. or one cup, 250 ml.) are very beneficial. Avoid drinking large quantities of juices. One or two small glasses are enough. Juicing can also be useful to break a fast. If you do a temporary, cleansing juice diet, don't drink too much juice — a few glasses a day at the most — in addition to water. If you drink more sweet juice (fruit or carrot), you'll bring excess sugar into the body. If you drink too much vegetable juice (celery, parsley, etc.), you'll bring excess toxins into the body. Some vegetables contain many toxins that can be perceived in their bitter taste. This is not a problem when we eat them because we won't be tempted to eat too much. The toxins are buffered by fiber and saliva and the time it takes to eat the whole food. But when juiced, these toxins are concentrated and taken quickly. Anyway, these green juices, unless mixed with fruit juices, are not very tasty. I recommended them strongly in my book, *The Sunfood Cuisine*, but my understanding at the time was different. You can drink pleasant mixtures such as celery and apple, but anything that tastes bad, such as pure green juice, should be avoided. In all cases, only consume one or two small glasses of vegetable juice. The rest will be an absolute waste.

SMOOTHIES AND WHOLE FOOD

Blended smoothies are great for getting a concentrated meal that's ready in a minute. You can combine a bunch of fruit with some water, maybe add some dates and create a tasty smoothie that can be enjoyed anytime as a meal. This is better than juice because you get the fiber, which is an essential nutrient. The fiber in fruits and vegetables is there for many reasons. Nature didn't provide us with juice. And "wholesome" means just that: whole. Whole foods are foods as they are found in nature, with nothing added or removed. In our modern world, juicing is a concession that must be used in moderation. Sticking to whole foods is always better.

THE RAW SOUP

The raw soup, which is actually a blended vegetable smoothie, is an excellent raw meal that can be prepared in minutes. For some reason, I really enjoy this during the winter. To make a raw soup, start by blending some tomatoes or cucumbers, and add a variety of vegetables: celery, green vegetables, sunflower sprouts, etc. Cream it up with some avocado. You can add one tablespoon of hemp seed oil or olive oil. As a seasoning, use some home-made, dehydrated vegetable powder. I have created a little raw soup recipe booklet — see the end of this book for ordering information.

CARROT JUICE

Proponents of carrot juice are numerous. A lot of books have been written hailing carrot juice as a miracle food — a cure for every disease. On the other hand, other authors have accused it of the worst calamities (raising the blood sugar, causing hypoglycemia) because of its high sugar content. Personally, I have nothing against carrots. No one ever showed me sufficient proof that carrots could be dangerous to our health. No. Carrots are a perfectly respectable root vegetable. But I agree that drinking large quantities of carrot juice is detrimental. But the same goes for any juice: apple, orange, or even kale juice. All the benefits attributed to carrot juice could be surpassed by a simple diet of fruits and vegetables.

"So, Fred, can I still drink an occasional glass of carrot juice?"

Of course! Why not? But drink a small glass, not a quart. More would be pure excess.

19

THE 100% RAW DIET

Fanaticism takes most of the credit for dietary self-sabotages. It is through fanaticism that people loose their sense of reality and cannot judge the results of their actions objectively. Obsessed with the idea that a completely raw diet is the ultimate, raw-foodists sometimes forget the bigger picture.

Although 100% raw eating is optimal, the way some raw-foodists eat is not necessarily healthy, as we have seen. It's not simply because a meal is raw that it's going to be healthier. A 100% raw diet works when done correctly, but it cannot be done in any which way.

I have met many people who were raw-foodists for 2 or 3 years and then went back to eating the SAD (Standard American Diet) because of constant cravings and dissatisfaction. Wouldn't it have been better to have figured out something more sustainable, instead of going back to meat and bread?

WHO IS REALLY 100% RAW?

A friend of mine travels North America teaching people about the raw diet. He told me that after meeting dozens of people who had eaten a raw diet for many years, he had never met anyone who had been 100% raw for a long period of time (over 20 years). At some point, they all either went back to some cooked foods, or experimented with cooked foods, or ate cooked foods thinking they were raw.

Do you know anyone that has eaten only fresh fruits and vegetables for over 20 years and never once tasted a bite of cooked food, or eaten a recipe that contained a cooked ingredient (Bragg's Liquid Aminos, dried herbs, spices, carob powder, etc.), never once succumbed to the temptation of a few (non-raw) cashew nuts, or eaten dried fruits or nuts from the health food stores that had been heated and frozen?

RAW AND UNHEATED: NOT THE SAME

There is big difference between what is raw and what is merely unheated . According to the dictionary, raw, in addition to meaning "uncooked" means "not processed, purified or refined." Raw food is food in its natural state — whole fruits, vegetables, nuts and seeds. This is my definition of "raw." Nut butters, oils, vegetable powders, sauces, etc., could be *unheated,* but are they truly "raw"?

I don't consider the following foods to be truly raw, that is, completely unadulterated, even though some of them are technically unheated: most store-bought nuts and seeds, dried foods, oils or coconut butter, tahini, carob powder, nut butter (any type), dried spices, herbs and frozen fruit.

How many raw-foodists eat foods from the list above? Most of them, I will say. So why make a big fuss about 100% raw when a lot of the foods they hail as raw are not? Instead of constantly worrying about raw, think in terms of health. Ask yourself: Is this really healthy for me? Do I feel great after eating it? Is it a specific food for humans? Is this a fruit? Is this a vegetable? Is this easily digestible?

So really, when we talk about a 100% raw diet, we really mean 98-99% raw. We mean a diet that avoids heating foods, but unless one only eats only fresh raw fruits, vegetables, nuts and seeds — without making any exception, this diet is not truly 100% raw.

RAW IS NOT THE ONLY CRITERION

We have to have some common sense, and be aware that not everything raw is better than anything cooked. I consider cooked vegetables to be easier on the body than nuts and seeds in fair amounts. For example, you could make a large salad and serve it with cooked broccoli and carrots and it will be easier to digest than if you mix a bunch of nut butter with it.

Though I recommend a vegetarian diet, I consider the "junk food" category (pizza, chips, fried foods, coffee, ice cream, pastries) to be worse than meat. So a piece of chicken with a salad is not as bad as a slice of pizza with a salad.

Our ideal foods are fresh fruits and vegetables — fresh produce (including fresh nuts and seeds). They are our true natural foods. Everything else is a concession to the artificial world we live in.

A RATIONAL APPROACH

It is impossible to be 100% right or 100% strict. Beware of militant proposals. I knew people who, after years of eating a 100% raw diet, were dreaming of eating huge chocolate cakes. But if someone has dreams like that, it means he is not satisfied with what he eats. I hope that, by reading this book, you get good ideas on how to balance your diet and make it more satisfying and sustainable.

Many raw-foodists either cheat or make mistakes. What types of mistakes can be made on a 100% raw food diet? They are numerous and have been reviewed in this book. Here is a summary:

COMMON MISTAKES MADE BY RAW-FOODISTS

- Use of salt, condiments, spices
- Eating too many avocados
- Eating too many nuts
- Constantly worrying and thinking about food
- Drinking large quantities of juices
- Eating honey
- Eating a raw diet except for drinking coffee or tea.
- Eating lots of sprouted beans and grains
- Sleeping not enough or at irregular hours and thinking that because they are raw-foodists, they will escape the consequences
- Paying no attention to digestion, dismissing hygienic food combining and eating complex mixtures.
- Overeating greens by dulling the taste with gourmet salads
- Overeating acid fruit
- Overeating dried fruits
- Eating a lot of oil

Some 100% raw-foodists don't cheat and don't make these mistakes. They feel balanced and healthy. Superb! Keep on. I would not recommend any changes to these people. I am proposing a raw diet — all-raw, or close to it, done correctly — but I think it's time to get rid of these fantasies that a 100% raw food diet is the solution to everything, and that it can work easily in all cases and situations. The experience of many raw-foodists throughout the world proves that a raw food diet is very beneficial — but it's not the only factor in health, nor the most important, and it cannot be done recklessly.

It's not a sin to occasionally eat few steamed vegetables if you feel that you can't stick to a 100% raw diet at this point. Not all cooked foods are equal. Steamed vegetables are easy on the body and will not wear you down like other cooked foods (bread, pasta, meat, etc.) You can easily limit yourself to fruits and vegetables without going into grains, dairy, bread and meat. Steamed vegetables have helped me and others make the transition to the raw diet much better than complicated raw recipes, which, in my opinion, are "gateway foods" to worse things.

Is 100% RAW EASIER?

Eating 100% raw, or actually 100% unheated, may be easier than eating 90% raw. When we are ready and start to eat all-raw, our desire to eat cooked food goes away after a few weeks. That is, of course, if pay attention to all the factors I have reviewed in this book.

Although it is in the reach of almost everyone to eat an all-raw diet, some people may not have the health or the mental and physical constitution to do it right now. They will need a well-planned transition. A competent Hygienic practitioner would never recommend an all-raw diet to everyone immediately, in every single case. Diet has to be adapted to people's needs, not conform to an ideal.

20

BINGES AND CRAVINGS

The scene is familiar. You have been pure for many weeks. You feel great. You feel confident. But one day, you are tempted to try a piece of something forbidden. Everything goes well, of course, because you only ate a little bit — of cheese, chocolate or bread. But the next day, the thought is there, troubling and unwavering — that chocolate requires another sampling. This time, you eat a little more. You feel a little drunk with the excitement of doing something forbidden, like the teenager smoking in the garage. However, the third day, in spite of your best efforts, you fall and hard. An abominable binge of bread, chocolate, cheese and chips follows. And the worst part of it? You get little pleasure from it, but you can't seem to stop yourself. After that, it takes you weeks to get back on track — feeling morose, sick and angry at yourself.

BINGEING COMMON AMONG RAW-FOODISTS: AN OPEN SECRET

Bingeing is quite common among raw-foodists. When it's not with cooked food, it's with dried fruits, nuts, and combo-abombos. There are many reasons for this — partly psychological, partly physical. Part of it is out of a frustration, which arise from eating a diet we are unaccustomed to. Part of it is out of a real, physiological imbalance. Let's see what Mosséri has to say about it:

> It is deplorable that most hygienists only observe and expose the lamentable situation [of bingeing] in their followers, without trying to find the reasons or analyze the causes. "I was a small

eater," a poet told me. "But after switching to the hygienic diet, I became a bulimic overeater!" This situation is unfortunately very common and even almost general among our followers. Let us examine the matter and find a reasonable remedy for it.

There is the bulimia that affects those with psychological problems and the bulimia that occurs after dietetic mistakes. Armed with the best intentions, we often fall in the trap of bulimia, without wanting it and without being able to avoid it. We often find this situation nowadays among Sheltonians and instinctos.

The followers of the latter method take a plant laxative everyday — cassia. The foods eaten are rejected the next day in abundant stools and do not benefit the body. This is why their cells are constantly hungry and the person becomes bulimic. For those that are not aware of it, instinctotherapy is the new fad which consists of following our instinct when choosing foods, smelling them and tasting them, according to our desire of the moment, whether we are hungry or not. But before selecting foods with the sense of smell, often distorted, is it not better to wait to be hungry? It seems more important to me. But the followers of this vogue eat without being hungry, according to their caprice. In effect, those who follow this method justify their eating nuts and seeds, meat and fish, on the basis of their sense of smell. But there are also Sheltonian hygienists who eat too many nuts and seeds. These concentrated protein foods are indigestible and rejected, *along with the digestible ones*, in putrescent stools the next day. We don't benefit from any of what we eat, which is why we are always hungry and start bingeing. Shelton used to say that an excess of fruit gives a small diarrhea in his followers. This is true when nuts and seeds are eaten, in the quantities he recommended, that is, a large handful (4-5 ounces). But if we never eat nuts, or eat them in small amounts, we never get diarrhea when we eat too much fruit. The reason is that nuts are so hard to digest that they end up weakening digestion itself and intoxicating the blood. Consequently, we must not make the mistake of saying that diarrhea is caused by an excess of fruits, when it is the nuts and seeds.

I have pointed out the main cause of bulimia in Hygienists and instinctos: the overconsumption of nuts and seeds in both and the eating of unnatural foods without hunger, followed by a daily laxative in the latter. We can see that the situation of the instincto is the worse of the two. Their bulimia reaches heights never known in human history. Imagine: 30

bananas at one sitting, or 20 apples and so on. The meal is capped off with a laxative, paving the way for reprise of the bizarre routine the next day...

À la Recherche d'une Santé Parfaite.

Mosséri points to the over-consumption of nuts and seeds as being the main reason why hygienists and instinctos become bulimic and indulge in binges. Obviously, it applies to raw-foodists as well. I have found this to be true. Eating a large amount of nuts feeds the body very little. Rather, it intoxicates it and fosters under-nutrition. The next day we are hungry, craving anything. This has been confirmed by the experiences of hundreds of people. However, there are many causes to this bulimia, not just the abuse of nuts and seeds. Overeating is a common cause. When eating large meals, little is digested and we are hungry because the body was not well fed. It's a vicious cycle that must be broken.

THE RIGHT ATTITUDE

We must cultivate the right, balanced attitude towards food. Moderation is possible in everything — even when going off-track. There are levels of dietary deviation: the small ones and the big ones. Most raw-foodists and natural hygienists seem to fall for the big ones. When they stray off their diet, you better watch out. They are like monsters unleashed! In their minds, a calming monologue may be going on to justify their excesses: "You can fast tomorrow" "You already went too far, you might as well enjoy it" "If I'm going to crash, I may as well burn." "It's not so bad, people eat like that every day," and so on.

Most of us have gone through these binges. Perhaps they are necessary to help us understand the damage caused by our previous diet. But the main problem caused by these indulgences is that they upset our instinct, our balance (which is restored slowly) even if we make only regular, "tiny exceptions." After that, we stop getting pleasure from unseasoned, natural foods, and start looking to spices and stimulants to excite our confused palate.

CRAVINGS

Cravings are of another nature. Cravings may lead to binges, but binges do not necessarily follow cravings. Binges may follow a simple taste of food, as described in the beginning of this chapter.

Cravings are a conscious, physical or psychological desire for a particular food or substance. They are often a withdrawal symptom and do not reflect physiological need. For example, an ex-smoker may feel a craving for cigarettes, which cannot be mistaken for a real need by the body. A coffee drinker, after giving up coffee, will crave coffee for a while until the body has detoxified all the poisons from coffee. Similarly, when giving up salt, bread, spices, pasta, meat, etc., the body may crave these substances for a period, during which temptation must be resisted with great will at all cost. But nobody needs these substances.

Psychological cravings are different — they may appear in an ex-coffee drinker, for example, after years of abstinence, simply by entering a coffee shop and smelling coffee. At this point, the mind becomes entranced by old images and all the associations it made with coffee. Basically, one has to snap out of the trance, recognize that the environment is triggering this desire and either dismiss it in the midst of the environment or, if it is too strong, leave.

Physiological cravings can occur in cycles. You can be free from them for a while, and then they can hit you with an attack!

However, after a few months on a healthy diet, it is not normal to be constantly feeling these cravings. In these cases, I attribute it to poor nutrition and a deranged assimilation, which is usually caused in raw-foodists, by anyone of these: an excess of nuts, dried or sweet fruit, salt intake, eating without hunger, the use of spices, etc.

Many people have never become completely balanced on a strict raw-food diet. After a few years, they still crave cooked food and sometimes fall into avocado, dried fruit, or cashew binges. Or this dissatisfaction can also be manifested in the constant desire for the new cleanse, that will ultimately free them from their "cooked-food cells." They go on liver cleanses, herbal intestinal cleanses, parasite flushes and other questionable attempts to improve their health and energy levels. But the true reasons for this compulsion have been unmasked throughout this book.

21

WHEN TO EAT

The following article is translated from Albert Mosséri's book, "À la Recherche d'une Santé Parfaite" (The Quest for Perfect Health)

"Those who adopt the hygienic diet start, with the strongest of wills, to modify their eating habits. They were used to eating small quantities of concentrated foods which, as we often say, fill us up. Being difficult to digest, they stick to the stomach for hours. These foods are bread, rice, cereals in all forms (croissants, granola, cakes, pasta, etc.). The new, hygienic eater replaces them with similar quantities of foods that digest easily and leave the stomach in little time, like fruits and vegetables (raw or cooked). So one or two hours after such a meal, these people experience an empty stomach. They take this for 'hunger,' especially if they are not used to eating large quantities of these new foods.

"Confused by this "hunger," which occurs outside of the fixed meal schedule, and getting poor advice from those who tell them not to eat between meals, they feel guilty about wanting to eat and are tormented by this persistent hunger. Then they jump on all the forbidden foods and eat them in large quantities.

"A lady recently told me that she has a small stomach and that she cannot eat a lot of fruit or raw vegetables at one sitting. One hour after such a meal, she is hungry. It is normal. Should she wait many hours to eat at "meal time"? No. She must eat again, even if the number of meals reaches seven a day, as long as she waits for hunger each time.

"In all my previous writings, and for more than thirty years, I have followed the pioneer hygienists, especially Shelton, who recommended two meals a day. However, I now realize that this has been a mistake. In fact, it's the hard-to-detect mistake so many eccentric natural hygienists make.

"Even women who are afraid of gaining weight should know that fruits and vegetables will not make them become obese, as long as they are eating nothing else, and especially, as long as they wait each time for acute hunger, to eat or just to nibble. They can thus nibble five to seven times a day, without eating meals.

FIXED MEAL TIMES

Don't eat just because it's meal time. If you wait for hunger and are hungry at 10 a.m., for example, but would like to eat at noon with someone, well, it won't hurt you to wait for another two hours. It's not so bad to be hungry. We shouldn't avoid hunger like we would avoid a tiger. Hunger doesn't need to be satisfied at the precise minute. Most people literally fear to be hungry, as if it were a sign of poverty or a sin, or death would fall on them if they did not eat at the first signs of hunger. No one will think that you live in misery, in poverty and in lack if you skip a meal, or if you don't eat every hour.

Dr. Virginia Vetrano

"She's right. So many people are afraid of hunger, as if it were a sign of imperative and urgent need.

"On the other hand, I'm noticing that Dr. Vetrano still talks, like Shelton, of skipping a meal. But I reject the idea of fixed meal times. I repeat that, in my opinion, it's better to wait for hunger than to skip a meal. The first injunction is negative and frustrating, whereas the second is positive and hopeful.

"Two remarks have to be made. Firstly, if we are occupied when we feel the first signs of hunger, we don't even notice it. Secondly, concerning certain, very emaciated persons in a state of undernourishment, the first sensations of hunger are accompanied by an extreme weakness — a faint sensation. These people must eat something immediately. For this, they must always carry some food with them, in case they leave their house. For example, ladies can put a few figs or dates in their purses.

CAN WE EAT AT NIGHT?

"Hunger is rarely felt at night, with some exceptions, such as during a long fast or in cases of undernourishment. It follows that we should never eat late at night. However, a fast can be broken at anytime, including during the night, with a piece of fruit. Those in a state of undernourishment can also eat a piece of non-acid fruit at night.

"Stomach digestion cannot properly continue at night. At night, all the muscles of the body loosen up, including the stomach. The consequence is that the stomach cannot energetically mix foods taken during the night. It is the same for the various glands that must secrete the digestive juices: at night, they rest.

"There is a basic rhythm — day and night — that must be respected in our lifestyle. It is the same for plants. If we water them at the wrong moment or don't water them when they need it the most, they wither away.

"For human beings, night is meant for catabolism and elimination, whereas the day is for anabolism and digestion. These functions should not be inverted by transforming day into night and the other way around.

"Hunger can announce itself early in the morning or many hours after waking up. We must wait for it before eating."

22

SPECIFIC AND NON-SPECIFIC FOODS

FRUIT

Like orangutans, bonobos and chimpanzees, humans are frugivores. A frugivore is fruit eater. Being a frugivore doesn't mean eating only fruit. All these noble animals include green vegetables, as well as nuts and seeds in their fruit-based diets.

Some say that fruit-based diets are dangerous because of the high amount of sugar they contain. They recommend a calorie-rich diet based on fatty, protein-rich or starchy foods. Fruit is also a source of calories (energy) in the form of simple sugar, which some people confuse with harmful, refined sugar. Let's look at the different possible sources of energy and decide what type of food should form the basis of our diet.

A high-fat diet will leave one tired all the time because fat is difficult to digest. The digestion of fat also creates many acids in the body. A high-protein diet is even more dangerous since the putrefaction of proteins during digestion is common. It will poison the body and lay the foundation for cancer. For these reasons, almost no modern health specialist will recommend a fat-based or protein-based diet. Sometimes protein-based diets (i.e., the Atkin diet) are recommended to loose weight. But almost no one recognizes this type of diet as healthy.

The experts generally recommend high-carbohydrate diets. Starch-based carbohydrates include potato, bread, pasta, etc. The advantage to these foods is that they provide energy in the form of complex sugar while being low in fat, while simultaneously being sufficient in protein. The problem is that grains tend to predominate in these diets. As we have learned, grains are not meant to be eaten by human beings. A grain-based diet will acidify the system as these foods are not alkaline-forming. A high-starch diet can work if it consists of cooked root vegetables such as potatoes, yams and manioc — all of which are alkaline forming.

When we eat complex carbohydrates (starch), the body must convert the starch into simple sugar. So ultimately, we get energy from simple sugars. Fruit is rich in a special type of simple sugar, fructose. This sugar is metabolized easily. Fruit is also alkaline-forming and richer in nutrients than starchy foods. In addition, fruit can be eaten raw, so all the vitamins, minerals, and enzymes stay intact and are not destroyed by cooking.

We can draw the conclusion that fruit should dominate in the diet. Fruits are rich in vitamins, but sometimes low in certain minerals, which are abundant in vegetables. This is one of the reasons why vegetables, especially the green leafy ones, are also essential. Of course, a lot of fruits are not particularly sweet: tomato, cucumber, pepper, squash, etc. (I call them fruit-vegetables and although they are fruits botanically, I classify them as vegetables.) We should not eat sweet fruit all day long, but change in the evening to vegetables.

The fruit we get in stores is also quite different from fruit found in the wild. Store-bought fruit has been hybridized to appeal to the tastes of our ancestors — and the increasingly perverse tastes of the modern masses. This fruit contains more sugar, less fiber, fewer enzymes, minerals and vitamins. Often they have been picked unripe. Even so, they are better than the rest of the foods found in a supermarket.

Some people think we should avoid hybridized fruits, such as pineapple, bananas, seedless grapes and Fuji apples. However, they don't acknowledge that the other commercial fruits, such as mangoes (the bestselling fruit in the world), cherimoyas, and papayas are also hybridized. Not only those, but all vegetables and everything else in the store, for that matter. So we shouldn't eat anything? I think it is legitimate to want to get genuinely natural, organic produce. But we must not make a religion out of this. People are not sick because they eat seedless watermelon. They don't get cancer because they eat Fuji apples. They don't get heart disease because they eat seedless grapes every morning. How about some common sense?

GREEN VEGETABLES

All frugivorous creatures eat green leaves and other vegetables. Green leaves are rich in minerals, while fruits are rich in vitamins. Green leaves includes cabbage, lettuce, kale, parsley and spinach, among thousands of others. The daily salad (see Appendix 2) is a delicious way to incorporate these foods in the diet. Otherwise, they can simply be eaten with avocados or tomatoes or blended into a raw soup.

Although I think that green vegetables are important, there's no reason to get obsessive about it. You can skip a few days and eat only fruit, fruit-vegetables and root vegetables. Sometimes we don't always feel like eating a lot of salads. It's better to listen to our body than to try to follow some rule that someone made up somewhere.

Salads and green vegetables are especially important for young children, pregnant and lactating women. They should try to eat them every day in good quantities. Children should be taught from an early age to eat their salads. Welcome their participation in the salad making — it's the best way to get them to eat well!

All sorts of succulent green vegetables — bitter, savory, sweet or mildly spicy — may be incorporated in raw soups, or blended salads. (see Appendix 2)

FRUIT-VEGETABLES

A lot of fruits are not very sweet, such as cucumbers, tomatoes, squash, zucchini and bell pepper. They are all excellent foods to eat at any time of the day. Tomatoes, however, must be taken in moderation, due to their high oxalic acid content. (See Appendix 1)

ROOT VEGETABLES

Root vegetables include carrot, parsnip, Jerusalem artichoke, potato, sweet potato, yam, manioc and celeriac. They are all excellent. Some of them can be eaten raw, while others, the more starchy ones, will be more digestible lightly steamed. Starchy root vegetables cannot be compared to starchy grains. They have none of their associated problems. There are several tribes that live mainly on cooked root vegetables and are in excellent health: no dental problems, no diabetes, etc. But these diseases appear automatically in these people as soon as bread and other civilized foods are introduced. Cooked starchy roots are superior to grains and may comprise 10-25% of the diet during transition. When everything is eaten raw, then all the less starchy roots can be used. Celeriac is especially good raw.

NUTS AND SEEDS

In chapter 4, you were warned against eating nuts and seeds in excess. This is certainly a common mistake many raw-foodists make. This being said, it doesn't mean that nuts and seeds shouldn't be eaten. They are part of our natural diet. Nuts found in the wild are delicious, seasonal foods; and the nuts cultivated today are not so far from their wild ancestors.

I have noticed that some people seem to fare better with nuts and seeds, while some can exclude them entirely without problems. Others will have to avoid them entirely for a long period of time, until their digestion improves. At some point, they can start eating them in very small quantities.

I warn against cashews, pistachios, and peanuts. According to Dr. Robert Young, these nuts contain fungus. I don't know if that is true, but I have noticed that the ill-effects brought on by these nuts are more accentuated than with other nuts and seeds. I think we can eat them every once in a great while, but not often. The best nuts and seeds, in my opinion, are almonds, pecan nuts, walnuts, macadamia nuts and hemp seeds.

Soaking nuts and seeds helps their digestion. But I don't think it is necessary if we eat them in small quantities and not every day.

WILD PLANTS

Edible wild plants grow everywhere. Most of them are quite nutritious, containing an abundance of vitamins and minerals. They have not been hybridized and are freely available, strong, sturdy plants. For this reason, a lot has been written on the benefits of eating wild plants.

But should we think of wild plant as another panacea? Another miracle food? Should we eat them just because they contain an abundance of vitamins and minerals?

Many wild plants are very bitter and taste bad, even though they may be edible. Forcing yourself to eat them would be the equivalent of forcing yourself to eat a food that you hate, or taking a supplement or a drug just because an expert has made you think it is "good for you."

But I reason that nature gave us the sense of taste to be able to determine what foods we should or should not eat. No animal would ever eat something just because it is "good for it."

The strong bitterness we detect in many foods is an indication that these foods contain some poisons. This is why some people believe that eating a large quantity of dandelion greens will cleanse their liver. But in fact, the liver is actually cleansing the poison contained in the dandelion greens.

I don't mean to say that we should avoid all these plants because some contain small quantities of poison. We have a liver that can handle small amounts of these substances, as long as we rely on our sense of taste to eat the right quantity, and don't season or mix them with other foods to fool our palate. If these foods are, or become too bitter or unappealing, we should stop eating them.

Wild plants contain much more minerals and vitamins than cultivated vegetables. Precisely because of this potency, it is not possible to eat a lot of them. Small, regular quantities of edible wild plants are very beneficial. Eating them in excess is not.

Edible wild plants may be eaten as long as they taste good to you. If you find them too bitter, you shouldn't force yourself to eat them. Think about the child or the animal, who has not been so corrupted by our twisted ways of thinking. It will never force itself to eat something that tastes bad if it doesn't have to.

I found that some wild plants taste too bitter. At some point in my "wild experimentation," I had to realize that if I were a wild human, I probably would not have forced myself to eat many of these plants. Other wild plants such as purslane, young dandelion leaves, milk thistle, sorrel, and lambs quarter, have a pleasant taste.

You can live without wild plants. If your digestion and assimilation are good, you will get all the vitamins and minerals you need from cultivated fruits and vegetables. However, I think we can also benefit from including wild plants in our diet. Never force yourself to overeat them just because you think they are good for you.

DRIED FRUITS

I don't consider dried fruits to be raw foods, but I don't condemn them entirely. They are useful during the winter. Most people have a tendency to overeat them. This has bad consequences: gas, indigestion, frequent urination, digestive discomforts, cravings, and disturbed sleep. I recommend eating them in moderation at the end of a fresh fruit meal to avoid overeating. You need to soak all these dried fruits except dates. Otherwise, they are very difficult to digest. The quantities? Depending on the person: 1-5 large figs, 5-15 medium-sized dates, a handful of raisins, 4-8 apricots, etc. The best dried fruit is the date, which is not artificially dried, but naturally "dries" on the plant.

Commercial dried fruits are subjected to sulfuric fumes. This gives them a more appealing color and appearance. It enables the sale of dried fruits with a much higher water content, so the manufacturer gets more money per pound. The added sulfur makes these dried fruits toxic and acidifying. This is why we should always buy organic dried fruit.

FROZEN FRUIT

I don't consider frozen fruits and vegetables to be truly raw because freezing physically changes the structure of the food and destroys many nutrients. The odds of finding frozen fruits in nature are almost nil. Imagine a monkey climbing up a mountain to its icy cap with a bunch of bananas, dropping them in the snow to freeze, then coming back days later to eat them (with its Champion juicer). The main problem with frozen "raw" foods is that they are eaten cold, which is the equivalent of putting an ice pack in the stomach. It is almost certain to cause indigestion. If you happen to eat frozen fruit, like durian, wait for it to thaw before consumption.

MILK

That humans need to drink the milk of another animal after being weaned from their own mothers, is an idea so bizarre one has to smile. It is not based on anything scientific. Rather, it is the spawn of a well-planned, well-executed, decades-long propaganda campaign by the dairy industry. Milk naturally carries powerful growth hormones that are deeply disturbing to our bodies. It is also loaded with antibiotics, bacteria, pesticides and cholesterol. It takes 10 pounds of milk to make one pound of cheese, so this cornucopia of toxic elements is even more concentrated in cheese than in plain milk.

Contrary to the propaganda, drinking milk will *not* prevent osteoporosis. The 1995 *Harvard Nurses' Health Study*, conducted on more than 75,000 women, showed that those getting calcium from milk experience more fractures, compared to those drinking little or no milk. Another study done in 1994 in Sydney, Australia, showed much the same thing — higher consumption of dairy products was associated with increased fracture risk. Those who consumed the most dairy products doubled their risk of hip fracture, compared to those who ate less dairy products. Other studies have shown that high protein consumption is associated with an increased incidence of osteoporosis.

Animal milk is for the animal's young and not for humans. All species stop drinking milk after a certain age and we are no exception. But the milk industry tries to convince us that cow's milk is "nature's perfect food" and that we must never be weaned! It is indeed a perfect food — for baby cows! Nonetheless, raw goat's milk can be useful in the case of a human mother who cannot nurse long enough, for whatever reason. Vegan mothers who give soy milk to their children are mistaken. Soy milk cannot replace real milk for growing children because it is lacking in too many essential nutrients. It is also cooked.

Adults cannot digest milk well since the enzymes that digest milk stop being produced after the age of 7 or 8. Drinking milk past that age will lead to several health challenges. When it is fermented and clabbered (like yogurt), it is much more digestible, but still not ideal, nor is it natural.

HONEY

Honey may be worse than white sugar. It has very little nutritive value and contains many harmful acids. These acids disturb digestion, the nervous system and cause cavities faster than white sugar. Honey, raw or otherwise, is meant to be eaten by bees, not by humans.

I no longer eat honey, except maybe once every six months and then only a tablespoon. A few years ago I was eating a lot of honey (but still less than I see some people eating) during a period of a few months. It was raw, organic, and of the best quality. Because of this, I developed a few cavities. As a child I ate sugar and sweets, sometimes in large quantities — much more than I ate honey — but did not get cavities. My experience has been similar to that of many others: honey can cause tooth problems, and fast.

EGGS: A NATURAL FOOD?

Eggs have to be stolen from birds, so they are probably not natural foods for humans, although some serious researchers, like Dr. Gian-Cursio, see a lot of benefits in eating their yolks.

Personally, I am not attracted to egg yolks, so I don't eat them. But I'm not opposed to them either. Note that two egg yolks at any one time is the maximum that should be eaten. Egg white is dangerous, acid forming, too rich in protein, indigestible, and should never be eaten, especially raw. It will be better to give it to your cat or dog.

MEAT: NOT A GOOD IDEA

I have never doubted that meat, the flesh of animals, has no place in the human diet. I do not want to expound my point of view here, because most of my readers are already convinced vegetarians. My observations have led me to believe and I'm not the only one, that raw meat is especially bad — worse than cooked meat. I don't recommend it to anyone. But I don't recommend cooked meat either.

FISH: EVEN WORSE THAN OTHER MEAT

Fish is probably worse than other meat. It putrefies much faster. If you put a piece of fish near a piece of meat, you'll see that it decomposes much faster than the meat. The same happens inside your body. All marketed fish have already started to rot. Fresh fish doesn't smell bad. It is an especially poor choice given all the heavy metal contamination that fish contains — a result of water pollution. For these reasons, I recommend avoiding fish at all times.

INSECTS?

Some authors say that insects are part of the human diet, because all apes sometimes eat them to varying degrees. Apparently, some monkeys are especially fond of ants. Personally, I have never tried them and don't plan to! On the other hand, when I eat wild greens, I don't wash them and they probably have tiny bugs on them.

23

COMPROMISES

Inevitably, some people will admit, "Look, I really believe in what you say, but there is just no way I can do this 100%, all the time. Please tell me what other things I can eat that won't be as bad." This brings us to the topic of compromises.

The compromises I am going to list are just that: compromises. You cannot fully reestablish your health if you indulge in them often. Better to avoid them. They are for those who are not going to eat just fruits and vegetables, or at least are not ready for it yet. They can help beginners during the first few months of transition. They are also for those people who, for whatever reason, feel they cannot go all the way with the raw diet. If that is not the case with you, then skip this chapter.

WHAT TO AVOID

Avoid breads and wheat at all times. Avoid milk and cheese. Homemade nut milk can replace animal milk. Yogurt made with nut milk or soy milk are good transitions foods. Tofu is too concentrated in protein and is difficult to digest.

If you are going to eat grains, avoid wheat and other grains containing gluten. Instead, choose some of the alternatives sold in health food stores (pasta made with spelt, buckwheat, etc.). Rice is slightly less harmful than wheat. Think not that these grains are healthy foods. They are merely *not as bad* as wheat products and junk foods. Products made with sprouted grains are to be preferred, as sprouting changes the composition of the grain, and consequently makes them less acid-forming.

Most of what is sold in a health food store is not healthy, but at least you can find some alternative products without preservatives and or toxic chemicals.

OTHER COMPROMISES AND TRANSITION FOODS:
Tomato-based sauces without spices; pesto sauce without spices; unsweetened yogurt; fresh, unsalted butter; unrefined oils in small quantities (1-2 tablespoons); coffee replacement (not real coffee but a replacement made with toasted grains sold at health food stores).

Grains that are easier to digest than wheat, and that are gluten-free include quinoa, amaranth, buckwheat, spelt and millet. In their sprouted form, all these grains forms are even easier to digest.

If you feel incapable of becoming a vegetarian, then have meat twice a week, but not more. If vegetarianism interests you at all, keep reading serious books about it. Eventually you will know too much to carry on eating meat and you'll know enough to free yourself from it. Avoid fish because it is worse than red meat (contrary to what most people think).

If you eat junk food or a rich dessert, then avoid combining other foods with it and make the next meal a simple salad or skip it altogether.

IT'S A LEARNING PROCESS
No one I know is consistent, and it can take a lot of time to hone in on this diet. If you eat something toxic, don't be hard on yourself. Just observe. You are learning. Use the opportunity to watch how you feel after. If you live in constant apprehension of the effects of your still "imperfect" diet, your fear is upsetting your digestion and further undermining your confidence. As Shelton has said, "Those who anticipate trouble from their meal, who eat in fear and trembling and who are anxious about the outcome, will be sure to have trouble. For these things inhibit, to some degree, the normal operation of the nutritive process."

We all know there are other factors involved in health besides diet. Although it may be one of the most important factors, it is not the only one. Peace of mind is very important. We can choose to be satisfied with what we eat by not worrying about how it could be better.

24

ORGANIC AND SEASONAL FOOD

IS ORGANIC FOOD ESSENTIAL?

I recommend getting organic foods whenever possible. If you cannot buy *everything* organic because of your budget or your location, it is not a major problem. Some people think that they are going to be healthier just by eating organic foods. Actually, they will eat exactly like before, except that they will spend more buying everything from the health food store. But eating organic food is not a major change. It is more a preventive measure. It is better to eat conventional fruits and vegetables than to eat organic bread, beans, pasta, meat and dairy.

Recently I went to an organic food fair where organic farmers were presenting and selling their products. In addition to fresh produce, I saw a lot of organic coffee, organic wine, organic bread and organic meat. In fact, the organic fruits and vegetables only made up a tiny portion of the vendors' offerings. The food offered for immediate consumption consisted of organic hot-dogs, organic beer and organic soda!

I have found that many organic items, such as apples, pears, yams, and lettuce are either the same price or only slightly more expensive than commercially grown, but they taste much better. So I recommend always getting the staples organic. Locate a farm in your area and buy directly from them. Or join a CSA (Community Supported Agriculture) farm. This is a service that lets you buy a part of an organic farmer's harvest in advance. Then as items become available, you get them weekly at specified pick-up points or directly at the farm. You get the best produce imaginable at the best prices and you help an organic farmer in the process. There are tons of projects like this going on all over North America and Europe.

To avoid pesticides, molds and fungi, wash or peel everything that you can that is not organic. Wash thoroughly what you cannot peel. I recommend a non-toxic fruit and veggie wash that is specifically for this purpose.

SEASONAL FOODS

It is now possible to eat foods from all corners of the world, at any time of the year. I saw cherries on sale recently — in January. To my great surprise, I met someone who had no idea when it was cherry season in our hemisphere. For these people, food mysteriously appears in the supermarket and they have no idea where (or when) it comes from, nor how it is grown.

I see no problem in eating imported foods. In many parts of the world, it wouldn't be possible to eat healthfully without them. But there is a limit. At least stick to foods grown in your hemisphere. Apples and kiwis from New Zealand during the summer, or cherries and nectarines from Chili in the winter. In addition to being expensive and copiously sprayed with toxic chemicals, they usually have little flavor and are a gratuitous distraction from perfectly adequate regional foods.

Stick to seasonal foods without making a religion out of it. Prefer locally grown foods when possible, but don't try to avoid imported foods if you live in a cold climate.

25

EATING RAW IN THE NORTH

THE IDEAL

The ideal diet may be a tropical diet. Unfortunately, our ancestors chose less friendly climates to settle in. Most of us live in cold climates where a good selection of locally grown fruits and vegetables is unavailable most of the year. One hundred years ago it would have been next to impossible for a family in Canada to eat a mostly raw fruit and vegetable diet all year round. But now we get foods imported from all corners of the world. Why shun these modern developments? A healthy diet is now possible for all of us, in spite of the steady deterioration of the quality of our food.

If you can move to a warmer climate and build your own little paradise in the sun, I sincerely encourage you to do so and wish you the best of luck. But not all of us will be able to do this. Most of my readers probably don't plan to move to Hawaii, Mexico, Costa Rica, or Florida in the next few years, and I write my articles with this in mind.

The winter diet of northern raw-foodists will be different than that of those living in the south. We probably have to get some extra calories in dates, dried fruits, root vegetables, nuts and seeds, etc.

In the tropics there are also many delicious fruits that are unknown in the North, but that could form a large part of the diet. For the rest of us still caught in cold or temperate climates, we will do the best we can in the part of the world where we are with the foods that are available to us. It is possible to eat healthfully anywhere, and yes, you can live on a raw diet — even in Canada! I have done it, so I know it is not so difficult.

FOOD QUALITY

During the long winter of the north, local produce is scarce. Lettuce is often weeks old, as it has to be imported from southern farms. Thus it may be useful to buy or grow fresh, sunflower greens. This sprout, free of the seed, can actually be considered a green vegetable. You can easily grow sunflower greens in your home. Cut immediately before consumption, they are certainly the freshest and tastiest of winter vegetables.

HANDLING THE COLD

Many people complain about the cold. Many raw-foodists give the strange advice of eating spicy foods, such as cayenne pepper and garlic. However, these foods are toxic (see chapter 7) and simply create the illusion of heat, just like the man who thinks that liquor warms him, whereas in reality it does the opposite. When you eat cayenne pepper and feel "nice and warm," it is just your body activating its metabolism to reject the poison (capsaicin) found in cayenne pepper.

A common reason for "freezing" during the winter on a raw diet is eating cold foods. Fruit which is still cold from the refrigerator when eaten will make you cold — it may even give you the chills. So my advice is to avoid cold food at all costs during the winter. Pull from the fridge the fruits and vegetables that you will eat the next day. They need to be at room temperature when eaten. If you want to eat something straight out of the fridge, warm it up in warm water. For example, immerse a few apples in warm water for 10 minutes. Do the same for grapes, pears, etc.

Bathing in hot water greatly reduces one's resistance to cold. Warm water dissolves the protective layer of oil out of the skin, increasing the rate of evaporative heat loss. It also increases exposure, through pores opened by warmth, to toxins in tap water, such as acidifying chlorine. Instead, take tepid (slightly warmer than cold) showers.

In general, if you desire an uncommon internal warmth, feed yourself what your frugivorous body functions best on: raw fruits and vegetables and a little nuts and seeds. Human beings are ectothermic creatures. This means we generate our own heat internally by the normal processes of metabolism and activity. We acquire it falsely from the cooking flame. We need only give our organism what it normally requires.

RAW SOUPS

Raw soups are a great winter food. For warm variations, serve them in a warm bowl or slightly warmed from the stove. The blending process can also warm them up.

TROPICAL FRUITS VS. TEMPERATE FRUITS

There is some controversy over which kind of fruit is better, depending on its climate of origination. One theory states that tropical fruits are better than temperate fruits because our body is more genetically adapted to them. So papayas, mangoes and bananas would be better than apples, pears and berries. However, I have never found substantial proof of this. Those that wrote this may have observed the fact that tropical fruits are sweeter, and appeal more to the fine palate of the raw-eater than cold-climate fruits. However, we could also say that tropical fruits may appeal more to the deranged palate of the hybridized food eater! Indeed, a clever person could say that tropical fruits like mangoes have been hybridized for thousands of years, whereas cold climate fruits like pears have been hybridized for a much shorter period. We may like them better because they are sweeter, but that doesn't make them more nutritious.

My thought about this is that they are equally good. Pears, apples, peaches, cherries — these are all excellent and delicious foods, just as papayas, mangoes and litchis are. You don't always have to seek tropical fruits, but to vary the diet is enjoyable.

Personally, I enjoy the variety of fruits that Earth has to offer, depending on where I am and what's available to me. In tropical countries, apples are more expensive than mangoes and are viewed as exotic items. But now in northern countries, mangoes are a common fruit on the table, which wasn't the case just ten years ago. Many of the most delicious fruits are not well known: cherimoya, litchi, jackfruit, durian, etc. As people eat more fruit, more varieties will be available to everyone.

26

FOOD SUPPLY

On a conventional diet, we do not notice the quality of our fruits and vegetables too much, as they are cooked, seasoned and mixed. On a diet of fruits and vegetables, being able to find a variety of good, ripe fruits and vegetables is imperative. If we are satisfied with what we eat, we won't be drawn to try other things.

PRODUCE QUALITY

Although I recommend buying organic food, it is not always possible for everybody to get everything organic, especially fruit. Organic fruit in health food stores is often unripe. If you want to eat 100% organic, unless you happen to live in a raw-food paradise, you will have to say good-bye to a lot of delicious and nutritious foods, like mangoes, papayas and fresh coconuts.

Unless you have an orchard and a garden, you will have to do some shopping to get good fruits and vegetables. This usually means going to several markets, supermarkets and health food stores to get the best of each. Some countries and regions have better fruit than others, but in most large cities you can find enough stores to insure a quality supply.

SHOPPING AROUND

Supermarkets — We might avoid going to these, but often there's no other choice. And nowadays, many supermarkets sell organic food. In England and Germany, I could find organic food in every supermarket. Supermarkets often have ripe fruit at discounted prices.

Farmers' Markets — The best place to buy fresh produce. Outdoor markets remain popular throughout the world, even after all these millennia. Get to know the farmers and ask for a deal when buying in bulk.

Exotic Fruit Shops — These shops specialize in exotic fruit and fancy items. Their prices are not the best, but you can find good stuff once in a while.

Produce Shops — These are either hole-in-the-wall family shops or supermarket-like stores where most of what they sell is fresh produce, often at very low prices. Even though most of what they sell is low-quality, commercial produce, you will often find good deals on standard items and sometimes, on local and tropical fruit.

Middle-Eastern Shops — The people there are friendly and you will be able to find good prices on good food, such as olives, fresh and dried figs, dried mulberries, fresh dates, date paste, etc.

Asian Markets — Once I found out about Asian markets, I knew my life was saved. I could live in any major city, even in the North (I'm from Montreal!) and manage to find exotic, tropical fruit at good prices! And I learned to say thank you in Chinese.

Asian markets are usually found in the Chinatown of a city. They can be run by the Chinese, Thai, Vietnamese, or by the Koreans. They will usually feature similar products a raw eater can be crazy about: fresh jackfruit, young coconuts, fresh durian, litchis, etc. They usually have very good deals on more common fruits like mangoes, bananas and oranges and seem to get better quality stuff than other markets.

People in Asian markets are usually very helpful and, unlike most supermarket employees, they actually know how to select ripe fruit. If you want a ripe durian, let them pick, because they know better!

Health Food Stores — There are many types of health food stores, so you'll have to explore to find the best ones in your area. Avoid the so-called "health shops" that look more like pharmacies than food stores with all their jars of supplements and bottles of protein powder. Find those that sell *food*.

I found that most health food stores now have a good selection of organic vegetables at reasonable prices. The fruit situation is often deplorable. But still, you'll be able to get all the staples: apples, pears, oranges, grapefruits, etc. It's also at health food stores that you will find dried fruits and nuts, but it may be better to order them in bulk.

Health food stores may be tempting. After all, it's all healthy stuff, right? Wrong. Better to quickly reach the produce section, get what you need and get out of there as soon as possible.

Mail Order Companies — In North America, there are several companies that sell nuts, seeds, seeds for sprouting, dried fruits and fresh dates by mail. You will find a listing for some of these companies at the end of the book. In Europe, there is a company called Orkos that not only sells fresh organic fruit, it's *certified raw* and unheated and they can also get you the most exotic fruits you could ever imagine. For those with a capacious wallet, Germany is a never ending fruit paradise.

Farmers — Next to growing your own food, what could be better than buying it directly from an organic farmer? You usually get the freshest, tastiest produce at incredible prices. Ask at your local health food store where to get a list of organic farmers and CSA (Community Supported Agriculture) projects in your area.

QUANTITY

A raw-foodist needs 2 to 3 kilos (4-6 lbs) of fruit and vegetables a day, sometimes more. The average family doesn't eat that much in a day and many families don't eat that amount in a week.

When eating such large, but normal, amounts of fruits and vegetables, buy in bulk, especially for a family, in order to get good deals and to insure that you have enough to eat at all times. A common reason for sliding off the diet is that people run out of food — and then get tempted to eat the other stuff.

27

FASTING WHEN NECESSARY

We have learned what to eat. We have learned to pay attention to various factors, and we seek to eat the best foods, or rather those that match our physiological needs and cause the least wear to our body.

However, there are times when even the very best foods cannot benefit us. In our lives, days are not always the same. Sometimes we feel great, sometimes we have worries. Sometimes we are relaxed, but at other times we are tense and have a lot on our minds. Some days one could experience headaches, pain or even a fever. In these conditions, even the best foods will not be digested. They may ferment and poison the body, further complicating the situation. And so, just as we must know when to eat, we must know when *not* to eat.

MISSING A FEW MEALS UNDER EMOTIONAL STRESS
Shelton explains:

> Strong emotions like rage, fear, jealousy and worry, and all intense mental impulses, immediately stop the rhythmic motions of the stomach walls and suspend the secretion of the digestive juices. Fear and rage not only make the mouth dry, they dry the stomach as well. Pain impairs the secretion of the gastric juice. Not only do all strong "destructive" emotions inhibit the delicately regulated psychic [endocrine] secretion, but even too great joy will do likewise...

Worry, fear, anxiety, apprehension, excitement, hurry, fretfulness, irritableness, temper, despondency, unfriendliness, a critical attitude, heated arguments at meals: all prevent the secretion of the digestive juices and other secretions of the body and cripple not only digestion, but the whole process of nutrition...

The practice of having the patient miss a meal or several meals if necessary, has my enthusiastic endorsement and has been my practice for years. It is a natural and an instinctive procedure, where instinct is permitted to hold sway.

Many times I have observed angry and frightened animals refrain from eating until, after the passage of considerable time, these emotional states had passed off. I have seen cows frightened and abused by angry milk-men and have seen them cease eating and not resume for an hour or more after the milk-man had departed.

It is true that under [stressful] circumstances many civilized men and women who refrain from eating, find, indeed, that they lack all desire for food. But it is also too often true that many men and women will eat large meals under these circumstances. Psychic and vital hygiene demand that under conditions of emotional stress, eating should be refrained from. Every one of my readers will enjoy better health in the future if they follow the example of the young grief-stricken lady who, thinking that she had been deserted by her lover, did not eat for three days, saying, when the lover returned, that she could not eat and refrained from all food until emotional calm was restored.

The Science and Fine Art of Food and Nutrition

PHYSICAL DISCOMFORT, PAIN AND FEVER

Natural Hygiene gives us excellent advice, but it may be difficult for many to follow, when it teaches us to *refrain from eating when in pain, mental and physical discomfort or when feverish*. Those that always follow this rule are almost sure never to develop chronic illness, as they are always letting their body detoxify when it needs it the most. Shelton, again:

> Pain, fever and inflammation each and all hinder the secretion of the digestive juices, stop the "hunger contractions," destroy the relish for food, divert the nervous energies away from the digestive organs and impair digestion. If pain is severe or fever is high, all desire for food is lacking. If these are not so marked, a slight desire may be present, especially in those whose instincts are perverted. Animals in pain instinctively avoid food...

The absence of hunger in fever has been shown to be associated with the absence of hunger contractions. This should indicate the need for fasting. Any food eaten while there is fever will only add to the fever. The fact that a coated tongue prevents the normal appreciation of the flavors of food, thus preventing the establishment of gustatory reflexes and, through these, the secretion of appetite juice, should show the great importance of enjoying our food. The feverish person needs a fast, not a feast...

The body needs all its energies to meet this new circumstance and it requires much energy to digest food. Food eaten under such conditions is not digested. It will ferment and poison the body.

The Science and Fine Art of Food and Nutrition

THE WEEKLY FAST

Fasting one day a week for 24 hours is an excellent habit to cultivate. This allows the digestive organs to take a rest and greatly benefits our overall health. When we fast and miss a few meals, the mind clears and all moroseness disappears. We find our balance again. Even the best raw-foodists make mistakes every week that add to their toxemia. This is unavoidable in our complex society. Who can completely avoid stress, worries and negative emotions? There are days when we miss a few hours of sleep, despite our best intentions. Who never overeats? Who always eats when genuinely hungry and when free of stress and worries? And what about temptation?

The weekly fast helps us correct these mistakes, by giving the digestive organs a short, well-needed rest. We can all benefit from it — especially those that have a difficult time sticking with the diet. It's a wonderful opportunity for a fresh start each week.

The weekly fast enables us to find our peace of mind and tranquility. Life's difficulties are not as overwhelming when the stomach is empty. Calm comes back and discouragement fades away. Enthusiasm is reborn and hope comes back. All the miseries will then seem less important than they first seemed.

Albert Mosséri
Santé Radieuse Par Le Jeûne.

Fast one day every week, on the same day or any day that you're not hungry. Eat a light meal the night before at 5 or 6 p.m., even if this means going to bed a little hungry. The next day, fast, taking in water or not. It is not essential to drink during this weekly fast, as the body is already gorged with water from the day before. Skip breakfast. Attend to your daily activities. Skip lunch. If you have a busy schedule, it will be easy to fast, as you will quickly forget about eating as soon as your lunch hour has passed and you have to concentrate on the tasks at hand. In the early evening, eat a light meal.

Pick out the day you are the busiest, like a Monday, to fast. You can quickly take to this habit as eating is likely to seem like an interruption on this day. Or, you could also fast on a free day and spend time alone. This is a good way to get back in touch with yourself. The 36-hour fast is not recommended, because, according to Dr. Alec Burton, it puts the body in the "fasting mode," where metabolism is altered to face the reality of the lack of food. But the 24-hour, weekly fast puts no stress on the body — on the contrary, it greatly rests it — and it can be safely practiced by everyone.

THE OCCASIONAL 2-3 DAYS FAST

There are times when we may need to fast for 2-3 days to get back our mental and physical balance. Perhaps we have made too many mistakes: not getting enough sleep; working too much; eating too much or without hunger; or by eating unnatural foods. Because of this, we may be feeling headaches, pains or digestive disturbances. It may be the death of a relative or a great love that makes us lose our appetite. In these conditions, we should fast for 2-3 days drinking water, instead of the alternative of eating without hunger and poisoning ourselves in this way.

Fasting for 2-3 days without supervision is safe for almost everyone. When the need is felt, usually manifested by a complete lack of hunger, then we can confidently, and with relief, refrain from eating until our balance comes back. The short 2-3 day fast is a good way to let our body heal, recover and get a fresh, new start.

Stressful situations — exams, deaths in the family, financial stress, etc. — may require a 2-3 day fast. Those who "eat their worries away" are laying the ground for worse ones, and are suffering enormously in the meantime. On the other hand, those who fast for 2-3 days under these circumstances quickly find their balance again and the inner power to face the situation with courage, confidence, a rested body and a clear mind.

LONGER FASTS

Longer fasts are often necessary when facing more serious and complicated health challenges, or for those wanting to experience the deep rest and rejuvenation brought on by a complete fasting cure. These fasts should be supervised, not by a medical doctor, but by a competent professional hygienist who possesses both a good understanding of, and is experienced with fasting. Please refer to appendix 5 at the end of this book.

28

A PRODIGIOUS DISCOVERY

Many of my readers are aware of the benefits of fasting. By resting the digestive organs and the senses, the body has a chance of ridding itself of all its accumulated toxins and can restore itself to health. Fasting, in many cases, is probably the "fastest" way to better health.

However, there is a lot of confusion spread by various hygienists and naturopaths on what is the best way to fast. We hear about juice fasting, "dry" fasting and even fruit fasting. Some authors recommend that their patients walk five miles a day, which is very detrimental when fasting. Others give their patients their own urine to drink or various supplements. Some people fast for 40 days, while others fast for one day a week. Others fast a long time while going to work, or while keeping up with their daily activities.

Many people imagine that reading one or two books on fasting (usually bad ones) is enough to know how to conduct a fast on their own. But they don't know the danger of this endeavor. They have not learned proper conduct during a fast. They don't know how to interpret symptoms. They don't know that, in some cases, fasting is not indicated. And they don't know how to break a fast.

Ideally, one can go on a fasting retreat and be supervised by a competent, hygienic practitioner. But these retreats, in addition to being expensive, are quite rare and nowadays, they are often led by medical doctors who add many useless procedures and tests to the fast.

Albert Mosséri, the giant of Natural Hygiene, whom I often quote and whose work I have studied for many years, has refined the Sheltonian technique of fasting to the point where fasting is safe and effective for every one. Unfortunately, his work is almost unknown outside of French-speaking Europe. I am grateful that he has authorized me to translate it. Here is a chapter from one of his books on fasting.

A PRODIGIOUS DISCOVERY

"In 1986, I made a prodigious discovery in the field of fasting that forced me to revise my Sheltonian method. This is how I was led to make this discovery.

"A 37 year-old man came to fast under my supervision. He had taken 104 different tranquilizers for his nervous state during the past 14 years. As soon as a drug wasn't having any effect anymore, the doctor prescribed him another one, thus the incredible number of different tranquilizers he took. He wanted to cure himself without drugs of any sort, so he fasted for 29 days.

"Then he became tense, incapable of relaxing or sleeping and unable to drink water despite an intense thirst and an acute kidney pain. I told him that he could not continue this way, even though he still had a lot to eliminate. His tongue was still very coated, his urine dark, his breath foul and he had pains in the kidneys despite all the water he had drunk.

"He responded that he still had a lot of time and that he wanted to complete his detoxification. So I thought that the opportunity had come, for the first time, to make him follow a detoxification diet. Every time a faster breaks his fast, he only wants to leave and I can't monitor his tongue anymore. For all those that come for a cure, my greatest concern is to facilitate the reintroduction of food, in a manner that avoids all problems. I must ration the quantities each day, increasing them and change the types of food according to each case. I do all this while watching the various symptoms that will guide me in this process. I rarely have this chance. I was fortunate to have such a determined man in my care.

"Three days after breaking his fast, I entered his room to bring him a few small apples. He told me, "Mr. Mosséri, look at my tongue." It was charcoal black!

"It didn't take long to understand this surprise. I had already seen a few cases where the tongue turned black during a fast. But this man was eating again. Yet the color was not accidental. I had provoked it with this detoxification diet. I had restarted his elimination, the profound elimination of a fast.

"I also realized that I could have done this much earlier — a week earlier, at the 20th day of the fast. He thus lost about ten days, during which time his elimination was very weak.

"His tongue stayed black for a few days. Then it turned a mustard yellow for many weeks, before returning to a healthy rose color. At the same time, hunger came back — a true hunger — and the kidney pains disappeared. I then fed him a normal diet.

"I wondered if this case was an exception, or if it could be imitated as many times as possible with other fasting patients. Obviously, the half-fast had accelerated his elimination, but one case does not mean much. I needed verification through numerous, varied cases.

"I started again in the same manner with two sisters that came after the man. The very day after they broke their fasts, their tongues were coated brown. Since then, 90% of my patients develop a colored tongue upon breaking the fast and commencing the half-fast and the other 10% develop it during a second cure.

"This half-fast must, of course, be continued as long as the tongue is even a little colored. A black tongue shows that elimination has deepened, reaching into the cellular level to root out decades-old drugs and toxins.

"Other questions came naturally into my mind: at what moment do we break the fast and go to the half-fast? What quantities of raw foods must be given to the patients?

"Having observed it many times, I already knew that a day comes when a patient's weight ceases to drop. Only now do I understand why. As for the food quantities, with a lot of trial and error, I arrived at the actual rations, more or less according to the height of the person.

"In the classical method, promoted by Shelton, the fast is pursued with water in bed. But when the fast is continued, though the body ceases losing weight, elimination becomes insignificant and time is lost.

"When someone noted to Shelton that a faster was only losing 200 g a day and that the elimination barely continued, he answered that it was 200 g gained and that it was still better than nothing. He did not see that we could jump-start elimination instead of standing about, making no progress.

"When the fast is pursued at this stagnant stage, weight hardly falls and elimination barely proceeds because the body does not have enough vitamins and enzymes for it. The body has just enough to survive. As we have seen earlier, the body's reserves are imbalanced. There is always too much fat and toxins and too few essential elements. When they run out, we go to the next phase, the half-fast, and the tongue colors itself in 90% of cases. For the other ones, it will color during a second fast. I could not find out the reasons why. On the other hand, with the classic Sheltonian method, it is very rare that a tongue will color itself, even if the fast is pursued to 60-70 days.

"When the tongue colors itself (black, brown, mustard, green or beige), the half-fast must be pursued until the color returns to a natural pink. That is, until the end of elimination. Then, the more concentrated foods can be introduced. The tongue becomes pink at the same time that spitting stops, the urine becomes clear, the breath becomes pleasant and the headaches are gone. The half-fast can last for one week or many, according to the degree of toxemia.

"With this new method, fasting becomes easier, with fewer risks and problems. The fast becomes mathematical, precise, scientific and without blind spots or surprises. This important discovery condemns the long fasts as a risky waste of time.

"I called this second part of the fast that follows the water fast the *half-fast*. But in reality, it's an elimination diet, since two pounds of food are eaten every day, half fruit, half vegetables. But I preferred to call it the *half-fast*, to strike the imagination of the fasting person. Otherwise, he would be tempted to think that he's breaking the fast and that he can eat whatever food and in any quantities. He has to stay with the impression that he's continuing elimination and that his cure also continues, although in another, less intense form than the complete fast.

THE REASONS FOR THIS NEW METHOD

"Whenever we stop eating, elimination starts and is evidenced by a white tongue coated with mucus, a foul breath, a bad taste in the mouth, a loss of weight and other symptoms according to the individual. As the fast goes on, elimination slows down because it uses up the body's stock of vitamins and minerals. Depending on the individual, this stock of vitamins and other essential elements lasts approximately 7 to 20 days. At the end of this period, elimination slows down, as revealed in the following symptoms:

• Weight loss slows to 1-2 pounds a week, stabilizing about every three days. It was 1-2 pounds a day before. The loss of weight signifies a strong elimination of toxins and retained water, which are urinated. When elimination weakens, we don't urinate much. This stabilization of the weight is the main signal to begin the half-fast.

• Thirst disappears and drinking water is difficult. Before, elimination created the need to drink in order to dilute the poisons and expel them in urine.

• The coating of the tongue is lighter in color and thickness, and the bad taste in the mouth lessens.

• Other symptoms specific to each individual can also reveal a slowdown in elimination.

Thus, when these symptoms of the slowing of elimination appear, it must be relaunched by breaking the fast and replenishing the body with nutrients in the form of raw, natural foods:

• 500 grams of raw fruits, spread through the afternoon. According to the height of the person, this quantity may vary.

• 500 grams of raw vegetables and salad, in two sittings in the evening.

"These amounts should not be increased, otherwise digestion will take the energy needed by elimination and bring it to a halt.

"The patient should drink a lot of water between midnight and noon, because that's when elimination is at its strongest. If the person is not able to drink at least a liter a day of plain water, then we flavor it with lemon juice.

"The fruits that I prefer to give are apples, because they act like a broom in the intestines. Sometimes, a water-rich fruit, like melon or watermelon must be given.

"As soon as we switch to the half-fast, rekindling elimination, we must examine the tongue every morning before putting anything in the mouth. It should not be washed. Within a few days, if not a few hours, it colors itself black, mustard, or brownish red.

"The half-fast is pursued until the tongue is completely clear. It becomes pink and all eliminative symptoms (thirst, bad taste in the mouth upon awakening, bad breath, spitting, etc.) disappear. It does not matter if, in the meantime, hunger comes back or not, because this instinct is usually defective amongst civilized people.

"Since the discovery of fasting at the dawn of times by primitive men, this discovery in the health field is the most prodigious that has ever been made."

From the book: *Le Jeûne, Meilleur Remède de la Nature*

Appendix 1

COMMENTS ON CERTAIN FOODS

FRUITS & VEGETABLES, NUTS & SEEDS

Asparagus — Asparagus contains an odorous poison that is eliminated through the urine. To be eaten in limited quantities.

Banana — Usually a staple in the raw-eater's diet. However, many authors condemn them for being too high in sugar and hybridized. On the other hand, Doug Graham, a learned hygienist, recommends them as a staple food (5-15 a day!) in his practice with world class athletes. As far as I'm concerned, the last word has not been said on the subject.

Broccoli, Cauliflower — I don't think we get much out of these vegetables when we eat them raw, because of their strong cellulose (fiber). Still, they are quite tasty sometimes. Eat small amounts and chew well.

Carob — Carob is excellent. Raw carob pods are amazing! Don't bite the rock-hard seeds. Get them from Raw Health (www.rawhealth.net). Though carob powder is cooked (no matter what the package says), you can use it as a chocolate replacement in recipes. Those wanting to give up chocolate may use carob bars to help them. But read the ingredients: some companies still include cocoa powder in these bars.

Celeriac — I love this vegetable! It is a root vegetable found in some markets and health food stores. Weird looking. Peel it and slice the inside. Delicious raw, plain or blended in soups.

Celery — I've always thought that celery is excellent, especially the variety available in North America. It is salty, rich in minerals and very delicious raw. Sometimes we feel like eating something, although it's not genuine hunger. We could chew a rib of celery instead of reaching for a piece of fruit or something heavier. Celery is very alkaline-forming.

Cilantro (Coriander) — Has a wonderful scent and aroma. However, it's not a plant we would want to eat in large quantities on its own. Some people have reported a mild diarrhea after eating it. It wouldn't surprise me. Use in moderation.

Citrus — Eat these fruits in moderation. There is a limit to the quantity of fruit acid the body can neutralize. That is why you have to be careful when eating acid fruits. Don't think you can eat them in large quantities. The citrus fruits and pineapples we buy at the store are more acid than those that we would pick fully ripe from the tree or plant. Acid fruits are best eaten before other varieties of fruits. So if you are going to eat more than one type of fruit at a meal, start with the acid fruits. Acid fruits are best eaten in the morning or early afternoon. Avoid them in the evening and especially at night. The body is tired then and will have difficulty neutralizing the acids.

Dates — An essential survival food for hard winters and during expeditions to the forest, mountains, desert islands, other planets, etc. I get them from The Date People in California (PO Box 808, Niland, CA 92257. #760.359.3211), who have dozens of varieties. You can order 10 different varieties at a time and eat them like pralines. I have also found great dates at low prices in some Iranian shops.

Durian — A fascinating and delicious exotic fruit. Can be bought at Asian markets, usually frozen. In Canada we can also get them fresh, but they are quite expensive. Even though I don't like frozen fruit very much, I have to make an exception for the durian, because it is so incredibly good. At the store you can buy whole durian or packages of frozen durian flesh. Ask them to choose one for you if this is your first time.

Greens — All varieties are excellent, except those that are too strong-tasting or bitter. We should try to eat them regularly, but it's alright if we skip a few days.

Jackfruit — Ripe jackfruit is by far my favorite thing in the world. Okay, it's my second or third favorite thing. Anyway, it's too bad that this exotic fruit is not available except in Asian markets, Hawaii, the Caribbean islands, the South Pacific and Southeast Asia. Ripe, its flesh is bright yellow, with a very sweet taste and the flavor of Juicy Fruit gum.

Pineapple — Look for varieties ripened on the plant. They don't necessarily have to be golden, but can also be green. It just depends on the variety. They are quite acid, even when bought ripe. In the tropics, when they fully ripen on the plant, they are not as acidic. Avoid eating too much (see **Citrus**). A few slices are good. Notice that closer to the base of the pineapple, it's actually sweeter.

Potatoes — Some authors have vehemently attacked potatoes using lame arguments. But steamed potatoes are much better than bread, grains, pasta, etc. They can be used during transition instead of bread. I would like to see the world eating more potatoes and less bread. Potatoes are easy to digest, low in protein, but their proteins are of high quality. Potatoes are alkaline-forming. They have to be cooked, but they don't have the same problems as grains. While not an ideal food, they are still far better than most cooked foods, and even to many raw foods, such as complicated recipes and nuts and seeds in excess.

Spinach — Spinach contain a lot of oxalic acid, so we should avoid eating it too often.

Sprouted Beans — I advise against eating too many raw sprouted beans. Steve Meyerowitz, the Sproutman, who wrote many books on sprouting, says: "Although sprouting makes the large beans easier to digest, increases their protein and lowers their starch, they are still primarily raw beans. Quantity and regularity of consumption is the caveat here. One should not *regularly* consume *large quantities* of raw beans or raw sprouted beans..."

Tomato — You can as much as 2-3 medium tomatoes every day, but avoid taking more. Tomatoes contain some oxalic acid. I have known many people who ate too many tomatoes, sometimes 2-3 pounds a day and suffered some discomfort because of this.

SOME POPULAR FOODS AND PRODUCTS

Bragg's Liquid Aminos — This product is an unfermented, wheat-free, soy sauce. The company says it adds no salt, but its saltiness is the main reason people eat it. The manufacturer refuses to explain how it makes it. This is itself very suspicious. Anyway, this product comes from a factory, is *highly* refined, and therefore, has no place in the kitchen of a truly health-conscious person. Nature does not produce any soy sauce.

Chocolate — Chocolate is eaten as a food, but in fact, like coffee, it is a drug. It is made from cacao beans. In both its natural and roasted state, the cacao bean has a very unpleasant taste, due to the presence of several toxic alkaloids, including theobromine — a poison similar to caffeine. But camouflaged with sugar and fat, it is eaten all over the world and cherished by people of all classes. Chocolate is a drug, a stimulant and a non-food — a pure abomination. Replace chocolate with carob, or pitted dates stuffed with almonds. The most astounding chocolate substitute I ever had, which some think is actually better than chocolate, is made from raw olives! In a food processor, combine dates, carob and the sun-and-air-dried olives found directly beneath an olive tree for the greatest, raw combo-abombo ever.

Coffee — Coffee is a serious poison and a drug. It is blindly consumed all over the world by hundreds of millions of people, who are chronically stressed by the insane demands of civilization. In addition to caffeine, it contains dozens of other poisons. Caffeine creates a frenetic, distressed state of mind (mistaken for alertness) as the body mobilizes to neutralize and reject it. This activity is often mistaken for energy. In fact, coffee drinking drains your energy. It's like whipping a tired horse so that it goes faster — eventually it will collapse.

Coffee drinking is hard to give up for most people. Depending on how many cups you are used to drinking, you may experience light or severe detoxification symptoms. They rarely last more than 2-3 weeks. Hold on! Have courage! To forget the habit of drinking coffee, you can use fake coffee, a safer, grain-based substitute sold in all health food stores. There are many brands with different flavors. Coffee shops that serve soy milk will let you order a cup of hot, steamed soy milk. Otherwise, order water, orange juice or fresh fruit. By the way, both black and green teas are nearly as bad as coffee.

Hot Beverages — The habit of drinking hot beverages is so ingrained in our society that when people stop drinking coffee and tea, they immediately panic, like a child who has lost his mother in a crowd, and they desperately seek replacements such as: herbal teas, fake coffee, hot cider, etc. The truth is that we are not meant to drink hot beverages. Their heat greatly damages the tongue and the mucus membranes of the esophagus, stomach and intestines. They also interfere with digestion. Most herbal teas are made with plants that have a disgusting taste when eaten in the natural state — mint, camomile, etc. I classify them as drugs, not foods. Yet I understand that the habit of drinking hot beverages is hard to give up, so I suggest the following hot drinks as transitions:

- Hot almond milk milk with a dash of cinnamon.
- Home-made vegetable broth without salt.
- Hot water with lemon juice or orange juice. Optional: ginger (boiled in water) and a touch of maple syrup.
- Coffee replacer, also called cereal coffee.

Avoid drinking these drinks really hot. If they burn your fingers, they will also burn the inside linings of the mouth and stomach, which are much more delicate.

Miso — Miso is a highly salty paste made in a factory with cooked, then fermented soy beans . In other words, it's unmitigated poison.

Molasses — A by-product of the sugar industry, but often sold for its iron content. An obvious hoax.

Mushrooms — I don't consider mushrooms to be human foods. As fungi, their role in nature is to recycle certain elements. Mushrooms are poorly digested and rejected through the stools. But still, eating a few mushrooms (the edible ones!) once in a while is without consequence.

Nama Shoyu — I briefly used this unpasteurized soy sauce a couple years ago. But it didn't take me very long to realize it had no place in the human diet. Nama Shoyu is not cooked *twice*, but it is still made from beans, comes from a factory and contains a lot of added salt. I don't recommend it. The same goes for any type of soy sauce.

Peanuts — Peanuts are really a legume, but classified as a nut because of their composition. I think we can eat them a couple times a month, though some people have stronger negative reactions to them than regular nuts.

Seaweed — Most seaweeds come from a factory, where they have been tenderized and cooked. Some are less processed, like dulse. The main danger to eating seaweeds is the levels of contaminants, such as heavy metals, they may contain. Even the organic seaweeds that are tested for these contaminants may contain them in some quantity, even though they are "guaranteed" to be within "safe" levels. For these reasons, and the fact that most of them contain a lot of sea salt, I advise avoiding seaweeds or eating them sparingly.

Tahini — Tahini is hulled sesame seed butter. If you buy it, pour off and discard the oil that has risen to the top. That way, it will be a little less rich in fat and easier to digest. I don't recommend eating nut butters often, but once in a while, they are okay. How much? One or two tablespoons. More would be sheer abuse.

Tofu — Tofu is cooked soy milk coagulated into a bland, chewy bloc. However, it is too rich in protein and fat, and it contains few vital elements. It is not very tasty and is processed in a factory. It is not part of a natural diet.

Yeast — Yeast, yet another substance unfit for human consumption, is nonetheless popular as a supplement and as a seasoning in vegetarian circles. It complicates digestion by encouraging fermentation. The role of yeast in nature is to reduce plant and animal substances to the mineral state. It is not meant to be eaten.

Appendix 2

MENUS

Here are a few menu suggestions. They may give you some ideas on how you could organize your eating schedule. If you find something different that works for you, then go for it.

MENU #1

During the day: Drink water upon rising. Start your day. Watch for hunger. After it comes, relax into it. Eat a fruit meal with or without lettuce and celery. Watch for hunger again, then eat either more fruit or vegetables.

Evening Meal: Have one of the following, depending on your schedule and hunger:

- Avocado, or fresh, in-shell nuts, followed by greens and/or vegetables, or
- A large salad (see below), or
- A raw soup, or
- Nothing (some days you may not be hungry)

Cooked Options:
- An assortment of steamed vegetables with some lettuce , or
- A large salad with steamed potatoes, or
- A home-made soup without salt or oil
- A large raw salad combined with steamed vegetables

MENU # 2

<u>In the morning</u>: Drink water upon rising. Start your day. Watch for hunger. After it comes, relax into it. Then eat some acid fruits (oranges, pineapple, etc.) or other types of juicy fruit.

<u>At noon</u>: A large salad

<u>4-6 pm</u>: Have a fresh fruit snack.

<u>Evening meal</u>: Have one of the following, depending on your schedule and hunger:

• Avocado, or some fresh nuts, followed by raw vegetables and greens, or
• A large salad (see below), or
• A raw soup, or
• Nothing (some days you may not be hungry)

Cooked Options:
• An assortment of steamed vegetables with some lettuce , or
• A large salad with steamed potatoes, or
• A home-made soup without salt or oil, or
• A large raw salad combined with steamed vegetables

THE LARGE SALAD
A proper salad is a delight for the eyes. Arrange a few chopped, sliced or grated raw vegetables. Use young salad greens, lettuce, celery and root vegetables. I enjoy adding bell pepper, tomatoes, cucumbers or thinly sliced zucchinis. Top it off with a few seasonings.

SEASONINGS
• Black olives, desalted (see Tips)
• Avocado
• One tablespoon of cold-pressed oil such as olive or hemp seed oil
• Lemon juice
• Chopped parsley or cilantro (coriander)
• Chopped green onions (not the bulb but the green part)

• Garlic flowers mixed in sunflower oil (can be found in some health food stores)
• A dressing made by blending tomatoes with avocado and some of the other seasonings listed above

STEAMED VEGETABLES
When I say steamed, I don't mean the popular method of steaming vegetables in a basket over a large quantity of boiling water which gets thrown away. This method of steaming robs too many vitamins and minerals. The best way is too cook in a pot, without a basket, with a heavy lid, with as little water as possible, so that there is little or no water left at the end. Any remaining water may be drunk before the meal. Steam only till vegetables *begin* to soften. They should remain firm and intact.

RAW SOUPS
Start by blending some tomato, cucumber or another juicy vegetable. Add a little water if needed and slowly add celery, lettuce leaves and other green vegetables. You may enrich the flavor by adding lemon juice and dried vegetable powder. Cream it up with avocado. A raw soup recipe booklet is available (see ordering information at end of book).

DESSERTS
During the cold season, you can soak 4-6 pieces of one kind of dried fruit like figs or apricots and eat them the next day at the end of a fruit meal. They combine well with sweet fruit, like bananas, but not with acid fruit. Dates don't need to be soaked.

TIPS AND GUIDELINES
• A raw-foodist needs around 2-3 kilos (4-6 lbs) of food a day. To put things in perspective, 2-3 large apples, or 2-3 bananas are a pound. Older, smaller or less active people may need as little as 1 to 1.5 kilos (2-3 pounds). Athletes may need 5 kilos. While this may sound like a lot of food, keep in mind that a raw-foodist doesn't need to drink a lot of water. Most of the water she needs is found in the juicy fruits and vegetables that she eats.
• Make a large vegetable salad in advance and store it in a seal-

able container in the fridge for a few days. That way you will have always access to a healthy snack and won't be tempted to eat unhealthy foods.

• Even though the types of food eaten are always the same, you can avoid boredom by varying the varieties of fruits and vegetables each day. There are so many fruits, vegetables and nuts to discover. Have you ever heard of: litchi, young coconut, cherimoya, Christmas melon, Asian pear, water chestnut, jícama root, bok-choy, durian, jackfruit, macadamia nut, longans or mangosteen? Have you ever tried a fresh fig? Or fresh, juicy dates? Try out a new fruit or vegetable each week, and start shopping at exotic markets.

• To desalt olives, the trick is to remove the pits *before* soaking them in water for 12-24 hours. Otherwise, soaking is ineffective.

• Avoid changing your eating schedule. Animals always eat in the same manner. If you choose to have the salad meal at lunch, have it then everyday. Besides harmonizing your body and your lifestyle, this enables you to notice how small changes in your diet affect you.

• Acid fruits are perfect in the morning, but are to be avoided in the evening.

• Prefer (non-fatty) fruit during the day and vegetables and fats after 4 p.m. This works best for most people, but of course, you can create your own menu based on your needs.

• Avoid eating late at night. Eat nothing in the three hours before bedtime.

• Eating one food at a time is ideal for digestion. Experiment with mono-meals.

• Some of the worst combinations you can eat are: *acid-starch*, such as tomato and potato, apple and bread; *sugar-starch*, such as dates and bread, bananas and bread, honey and oatmeal; *protein-protein*, such as avocados and nuts, cheese and nuts. The habit of eating nuts and seeds with sweet fruit (especially with dried fruit) leads to fermentation.

• Avoid eating when experiencing pain, fatigue, indigestion or fever.

• The weekly 24-hour fast is an excellent way to maintain your physical and emotional balance.

• Life is not a set of rules. Once you have discovered how to eat the natural diet in a way that brings you balance, health and energy, give it less attention and live your life!

Appendix 3

REPLACEMENTS & TRANSITION FOODS

REPLACE	WITH
vinegar	lemon juice
salt	dehydrated celery seasoning
spices	onions that have been cut up and left in the open air for 24 hours; fresh parsley, green onions, cilantro, dill, etc.
bread and grains	sweet fruit, baked plantain, dried bananas and dried fruits in moderation, steamed potatoes, occasional chestnuts, sprouted bread
chocolate	carob
coffee	fake coffee
milk	nut milk or soy milk
dairy yogurt	nut or soy yogurt
cheese	avocados
pastries, jams, candy	dates and other sweet fruit, soaked dried fruits with a little cream.

The ideas on the previous page for replacing foods can help you either give up something, or find a suitable replacement for certain foods. You will notice that some of the replacement choices are cooked. Use them in your transition from the vastly more toxic foods which they replace, and for those foods which you are trying to avoid.

Appendix 4

TESTIMONIALS

My comments in italics.

HAPPY ON A FRUITARIAN DIET

I have been eating 80% fruit since 1980. I am now a totally committed fruitarian, since September, 1999, eating only sweet and non-sweet fruits. The transition has been gradual, easy and permanent. I am 73 and my blood pressure has dropped from 200 to 140. I cleared all my prostate problems. Paunch gone. No more aches and pains. I am never thirsty or hungry. I do not have any body odor and hardly need toilet paper.

My six-foot body has gradually dropped from 87 kilograms to 80 kilograms. I want to be in a state where I do not have to cart around any more weight than I absolutely have to. I am not deliberately loosing weight or adopting any strategies to help myself, except to eat the best food I can — soft, very ripe, inexpensive fruit, which the average customer will not buy.

I puree everything to a pulp with a food processor and eat it slowly with a spoon. I am getting very good at making tasty mixtures. I am an apple cider vinegar and honey freak and put a drop of these in all the mixtures. I am letting Mother Nature, through my immune system, make all the chemical decisions. I believe she is very good at it.

Jo Mazzarol
Australia

This person was overweight to start with. Overweight people can benefit from a total fruit diet, until they reach their ideal weight. However, after that, they have to introduce salads and vegetables. I often receive such testimonials, but never from a person who has eaten all-fruit for more than a few years. Improvements on this diet would include leaving out the honey and vinegar, eating some greens and most or all of the fruit unprocessed and uncombined.

ENJOYING FRUIT-EATING IN ENGLAND

Thank you for your lovely magazine *Just Eat An Apple*. It arrived on a beautiful winter's day and I have been reading it, alternating with sun-gazing, in the rose garden of a local park.

Even in the middle of winter in England, the sun shines beautifully. In the shade the ponds are iced-over, but the fruit-eating sun-lover can always find a sheltered sun-trap.

I am enjoying a lot of local fruit — apples and pears — which are perfectly balanced for the autumn and winter seasons. There are still some wild apples to be found. They stand out on the bare branches of the trees, beautiful balls of color and life in the winter landscape.

One thing I often get asked, with reference to diet, is, "Don't you get bored?" Even on a mono-diet, each piece of fruit is unique and within each fruit exists a myriad of different flavors. If only people knew how to tune into a "simple" diet, they would find out how complex and enjoyable are the tastes within.

I find that keeping warm, on a fruit diet, even in English winter, is not a problem. It is a case of keeping one's vitality raised. If you breathe deeply and exercise enough, you will always be warm. Fruit also gives a wonderful flow of energy: you can walk all day and dance all night!

I found your magazine a wonderful accompaniment to a sunny rose garden and I enjoyed everything in it. Thanks again for enhancing a beautiful day with a lovely read.

Yours for peace, sun, fun and love,
Anne Osborne, United Kingdom

Anne is one of the rare near fruitarians. She eats some salad and celery.

RADICAL CHANGES

I just wanted to take this moment to tell you how wonderful I feel after having been on the raw vegan way of life (100% raw) since December 15, 1999. I feel like I have the energy of a 25 year-old and I have just turned 51! People are starting to tell me that I even look younger and that I no longer have that "always tired look." A by-product of this wonderful way of life is that I no longer use medication to control diabetes. My morning blood-sugar level is around 95 and mid day is 113. Since becoming a raw vegan, I have lost 83 pounds and I have never felt better.

Howard Fisher
Youngstown, OH

Those who are overweight are usually very happy when going on a raw-food diet. Their energy levels go up and they feel better every day as the weight drops. Thin or skinny people do not have the same constitution and tend to experience more fatigue during transition.

DOG DIET ALSO WORKS FOR HUMANS!

Not long ago I wrote you about the mostly raw vegan diet my friend fed her dog that lived beyond twenty years and endured no diseases. It occurred to me that your readers might want to know what I feel would probably be a better option for their dogs than regular dog food.

Breakfast: fresh, very ripe fruit pieces.
Lunch: Apple pieces mixed with dates pieces, date/coconut rolls, figs or other dry or semi-dried fruit to provide concentrated nutrition. You may wish to follow this with grapes.
Dinner: small green salad followed by extremely well cooked potatoes (that have been cooled and mashed with avocado, and chopped crunchy vegetables or fruit-vegetables. For example: pieces of celery and cucumber and small amounts of grated carrots.

Be sure to select genuinely ripe produce for yourself and your pets. If you buy mission figs, buy the darkest, blue/black ones you can find, that have the darkest red markings. If you buy dates or date/coconut rolls, buy the darkest brown dates you can find. Medium brown date rolls are usually not as bad as medium brown dates. When purchasing yams or potatoes, buy the darkest ones you see. Like bananas, apples and plums, potatoes that have dots are preferable because dots are indicative of ripeness.

In my view, very well done yams and potatoes are superior to soaked/sprouted seeds, nuts, grains, legumes, because the baked starchy vegetables are still much less mucus forming.

I believe a 100% raw vegan diet consisting of fruits, low starch vegetables, fruit vegetables, and avocados or olives is probably best. But only when one lives in a fairly pristine environment and can absorb and synthesize important health constituents from the elements.

Although I have practiced fruitarianism and raw veganism for extended periods, I now prefer this "dog diet" for myself as well! (Note that I often include well-cooked, low-starch veggies such as broccoli or zucchini with my evening salads).

In addition to limiting our intake of cooked products, in my opinion, our focus needs to be on reducing our consumption of mucus-forming foods, beverages and supplements.

Karen Schechet
San Diego, California

One does not have to live in a pristine environment to eat a raw diet. It can be done anywhere. Nuts can be eaten in limited amounts, as indicated in this book.

100% RAW

After a couple months of testing and questioning, I finally took the step of becoming 100% raw on fruits and fruit-vegetables. It is simply wonderful! My fibromyalgia has disappeared and my fatigue after every meal is nothing but a memory. My family used to make fun of me after dinner since I would become so terribly tired. This went on for years! After every meal I had to lie down and regain some strength to get through the evening! This is over, after only a week on the diet.

Another thing I notice is that my memory and brain-capacity have slowly improved — maybe I'll be able to go back to school and graduate. That would really be something! Thank you all for the good work and keep it up!

Lena Buhr
Sweden

FORMERLY OBESE

I used to be clinically obese and suffering from Hashimoto's Disease, a type of near-total thyroid failure. Raw veganism has nearly cured me of both these abominations. I am of average weight and approaching a healthy thinness (which has always been my ideal). My thyroid continues to recover more and more, to the point where my present dosage of thyroid replacement is only half as strong as my primary dosage in 1994!

Any idea that raw veganism is a "bland," "protein-less," "monotonous," or "anti-culinary" diet is sheer misconception. All my family now insists that I become a chef — a compliment I never received before in my cooking endeavors!

Jai Krishna Ramchand
Cardiff, CA

GOING NATURE'S WAY

I went raw for only six months, several years ago. I was introduced to it by my dad who had great results (got off his high blood pressure medications, had several cysts disappear, as well as overcoming his diabetes problem), although he did not maintain his diet. His health problems have come back and continue to get worse.

I had my first mammogram eight months ago — nothing was found. Within the last four months, a lump has developed that is just a little smaller than a golf ball. It scared me half to death at first. But at that moment I decided that I no longer had a choice if I wanted to reverse my health problems. I have chosen not to let the so-called healthcare professionals look at me. I already know what to do.

So I started my new lifestyle four weeks ago. I implement the "Ten Commandments of Health" that Dr. Lorraine Day teaches: proper nutrition, exercise, water, sunshine, temperance, fresh air, rest, trust in God, an attitude of gratitude and benevolence. I know that I will be able to heal myself. By the way, before my first experience with raw foods, I had severe migraines that made me sicker than I want to remember. Since my diet change of only six months, I haven't had a migraine.

Thanks for all the information on your website, www.rawvegan.com. I'll be checking back from time to time and referring others who want to attain health. I think your testimonial section is great support for other readers (like me).

Cindy Hatton

ARTHRITIS & THE RAW DIET

About two years ago I came down with a severe case of inflammatory arthritis, with pain in hands and feet and a badly spastic neck. The muscles there were as tight as a drum. In a nutshell: I went all raw and all symptoms went away; and they stay away as long as I don't stray into eating bread and pasta. Very coarse whole rye doesn't seem to affect me, but I don't eat much of that, either.

Since going raw, I have instructed dozens of patients in the same, simple course of action and have seen severe rheumatoid arthritis clear up in a matter of weeks. By far, the biggest problem for a person with rheumatoid is the drugs they are taking. Don't ever go that route! You're only wasting valuable time, because to get well you'll have to give them up sooner or later.

Carl S. Bosco D.C.
Coarsegold, California

LOOKING GOOD ON RAW

Ah, raw food. The "experts" will try to scare you. They'll say it can't be done. That it isn't safe. But it is, and ever so healthy, provided you eat a wide variety of foods. (And I've never taken a supplement, either.)

About 15 years ago, I read the book *Living Health*, by Harvey and Marilyn Diamond. It was their sequel to the best-selling diet and nutrition book of all time, *Fit for Life*. That got me started. The rest is history.

And, despite the dire prognostications of virtually everyone I knew (who are now mostly physical wrecks themselves), I'm walking taller than ever and still looking good. Oh, and did I mention feeling ever so good? And loving life!

Good Luck!
Anonymous

INFECTION AND ARTHRITIS GONE

I have been a raw-foodist for four months and have been cleansed from a two-year infection that the doctors couldn't clear up! Arthritis is slowly clearing up and I have more energy than I have ever had! I was just diagnosed with breast cancer in January and sure am hoping to get some statistics on eating apples to cure cancer. I've heard of cases here and there, but are there any clear statistics? It's already done so much in other avenues of my health. If anyone has other suggestions I'd appreciate hearing from you.

Jay Tudor
Sarasota, Florida, USA

As the historian Carlyle said, there are three types of lies: white lies, big lies and statistics. But for a book on the effect on cancer of eating a monodiet of sub-acid fruit, see Joanna Brandt's The Grape Cure.

FROM JUNK TO JAMMIN!

Most of my life I was getting by on a junk food diet: burgers, McDonald's, cheese, sodas, pizza, bottled orange juice and bread with an occasional banana or an apple. I always felt there was something very wrong and unnatural about the way I was eating, but the only veggies I had been exposed to were cooked, and I found them to be utterly disgusting. For this reason I never ate vegetables.

I used to play in the woods as a boy and pretend I was an adventurer surviving off the land. This is my earliest memory about thinking of raw plant food. It certainly didn't seem appealing to eat meat, especially if I had to catch it and prepare it myself, even though I ate meat almost every day. I'd find this disturbing that the food I was eating wasn't available in nature, and I didn't grow up where fruit trees were abundant. I fell for the protein myth just like practically everyone. I had problems through all of puberty (and before and after) with depression and lack of sleep. I had the cooked fooder weight lifter body for a while (some people think this is a good thing but now I see it as just being puffy). Eventually things were catching up to me.

Luckily I'd landed a job across the street from a Jamba Juice. I started drinking smoothies every day along with my taco bell, mac 'n' cheese lifestyle. I then graduated to wheat grass which led me to reading Ann Wigmore (*The Wheatgrass Book*) and discovering enzymes. If all my food was cooked, I wasn't getting any! I'd ordered *The Hippocrates Diet* by Wigmore and a guy in the health food store recommended reading the book *Nature's First Law*. I read it and became 100% raw virtually overnight. I had maybe 3 cooked incidents during the first month and I haven't had one since, over 16 months later now and am never going back.

I stopped smoking marijuana (it's cooked) shortly thereafter simply because I got to the point where it was bringing me down rather than up. My neck, back and hand pain has been greatly reduced, almost to the point of nil. My sleep patterns are healthy for the first time in my life. My depression is history. I've got great muscle definition now. More than ever, I enjoy eating, and I have no cooked cravings. Mostly I eat mono meals of fruit followed by leafy greens (whole or juiced). Its been months since I've had nuts, seeds or sprouts (just don't get the urge) but I eat fatty fruits (durian and avocado) and young coconuts regularly.

My skin and hair are healthier and softer all the time. Tanning is a breeze. My energy levels are growing all the time. I've gotten to the point where I'm pretty much high all the time as long as I've had enough sleep (and even when I don't, quite often). A cloud has been lifted from my body/mind and things are only getting better the more I detox the old. I no longer have "morning breath" even if I eat a lot of fruit and go to bed without brushing. Life is awesome. I recently met the girl of my dreams (yes, she's 100% raw) and am now heavily in love! I will definitely help every person I can (e-mail me if you'd like).

Brian (viihertz@rawfoods.com)
Dallas, Texas, USA

FREEDOM FROM ASTHMA AND ALLERGIES

I'm an Australian living in Holland now (for the past 18 months). I have been a "chronic asthmatic" all my life, and I have also suffered from hay fever and allergies.

It was one month after my arrival here that I experienced a particularly nasty case of hives (itchy red lumps all over my body, together with severe stomach pain), which the doctors here were at a loss to explain. They told me I was just acclimatizing to Europe; their advice was that I should get "more fresh air," and take paracetamol next time I get the rash!

After several bouts of these "hives," feeling physically worn out (not to mention the unbearable pain) I saw a different doctor, who recommended that I see an allergy specialist. Well, to keep the story short, I found out that I am totally allergic to milk — and all milk products (and have been all my life, the last 32 years!) The doctor also advised me to avoid all processed foods and foods with additives.

Meanwhile, I had also been doing research on my own, and found some terrific books at the American Book Centre in Amsterdam. I read about the Breath Retraining Program for asthmatics, developed by the Russian, Dr. Buteyko. He advises all asthmatics to avoid milk and all milk products, and also not to eat meat.

Well, Dr. Buteyko was completely right! A diet that includes animal foods such as meat, milk and eggs was making me sick. Suspicious of processed foods also, I gave up all the "convenience" foods I would normally be tempted to buy, such as canned food, instant soup, any and all kinds of processed food. This has meant avoiding 95% of the "food" at my local supermarket.

To my sheer amazement, within weeks of giving up all animal and "processed" food, my asthma just stopped! I would not wake up in the middle of the night, reaching for my "puffer" (ventolin inhaler) and becleforte (both immune suppressing steroids that accumulate in your body and eventually damage/ruin your adrenal glands). It stopped attacking when I laughed, or when I walked up the stairs, or ran for the bus, like it always used to. I was so amazed and overwhelmed, because for years the doctors told me "there's no cure for asthma," and I broke down in tears with happiness.

Determined to stay a vegetarian, and being concerned about getting all the right nutrition, I continued my search. It was while surfing the Internet, that I found your website (and a whole lot of other links).

Now I am totally free of asthma and allergies, such as hives or hay fever, and I've never felt better. I even play tennis, and absolutely love the fact that I can enjoy sport without medication.

An intelligent raw food diet is amazing. I am not 100% raw yet, but when I go back to Australia at the end of this year, I will invest in all the groovy equipment. For the moment, I am enjoying a diet high in sprouts (I grow my own), wonderful salads (with lots of yummy dressings made from my own homegrown herbs), raw fruit and veggies (especially avocado) nuts and seeds.

I am so impressed by the raw food approach, that I want to tell as many people as I can. The problem is, because of all the hype and advertising we are bombarded with in this modern world, the very thought of something so simple working so wonderfully sounds hard to believe. Now I am inspired to study nutrition in more depth, and get a professional education in health, so I can contribute to the movement that I hope will become the mainstream, in years to come. I am very glad I was open-minded enough to try the "raw" experience. It has changed me, literally.

Many, many thanks to all the raw-foodists, and people who create these helpful raw food information sites. You are such helpful, inspiring, courageous folk.

Angela Jackson
Amsterdam, Netherlands

MANY WAYS

It is interesting how people have so many different ideas on the same subject. I have also found that mixing greens with sweet fruit is a great idea. I just love green leaves and eat huge amounts. However I don't eat nuts or seeds and very rarely have any fatty fruits. The only fatty fruit I have is avocado. I find this diet ideal. It definitely keeps you very lean.

Pam
Perth, Australia

JUST SAYING NO IN ORANGE COUNTY

I have been eating raw fruits and vegetables for two weeks. I started doing it for health reasons. I am healing from a variety of conditions known in the medical community as Crohn's disease, nasal allergies, depression/anxiety, eczema, and acne. Prescription drugs I have been on for many years include Zyrtec for hay fever, Luvox for depression/anxiety, and Retin-A for acne. So far on this diet, I am feeling great and have lots of energy, clearer skin, and calmer composure. My acne has mostly cleared, and there has been a 75% reduction of oil on my face. My nasal allergies have cleared, and I have completely gone off my Zyrtec. I'm finally able to wean off Luvox after 8 years. So far the diet is doing wonders. I live in Orange County, CA. I would be grateful for any people in my area for support.

Anne D
Irvine, CA

You're surrounded! Check out the Raw Connections in our magazine Just Eat An Apple *for the tip of the raw iceberg there.*

WEIGHT LOSS, STRENGTH GAIN

I am a 99% raw vegan and am loving every moment of it. At 5'6, I used to weigh 150 lbs." Now I weigh 120 lbs with about 8% body fat. I love my new body and all the energy I get from raw foods. I am still doing lots of detox, but I am getting stronger every day. Love your website(rawvegan.com).

Werner Kujnisch
Dekalb, IL

CANCER

I just started eating this way two months ago after being diagnosed with cancer. Now I am feeling better than ever. Thank you for the information you have made available to us.

Claudia
Poulsbo, WA

LEANING INTO RAW

Your site is great! I became a vegan. Now I am leaning more toward raw foods. From everything I have read, it is the best choice for my health. I am having a hard time giving up processed snacks though. My family is still eating a SAD (Standard American Diet), but they support me. Thanks for this great website(www.rawvegan.com)!

Karen
Wheaton, IL

70% RAW

The information from this website is great (www.rawvegan.com). I have believed for a number of years how important it is to eat a raw vegan diet. I eat about 70% raw foods and I rarely get sick. God has opened my eyes to this truth and I thank Him for it. Hope everyone comes to see this marvelous truth.

Gregory Prisco
Mahopac, NY

Appendix 5

RESOURCES

RAW VEGAN
6595 St-Hubert, CP 59053
Montreal (Quebec)
H2S 3P5, Canada
www.rawvegan.com
info@rawvegan.com
The author's organization. Resources on healthful eating.
Publishes *Just Eat An Apple Magazine.*

NATURE'S FIRST LAW
P.O. Box 900202
San Diego, CA 92190
619.645.7282
www.rawfood.com
Tons of books, dried fruits, nuts, appliances, etc.

THE RAW LIFE
c/o Paul Nison
P.O. Box 443
Brooklyn, NY 11209
866.729.3438
www.rawlife.com
Books, videos and products on the raw diet. Paul Nison tours the
country giving seminars.

FRESH NETWORK
P.O. Box 71
Ely, CAMBS, CB7 4GU
United Kingdom
44.8708.00.7070
www.fresh-network.com
The Fresh Network is the main organization promoting the raw
diet in England.

ALBERT MOSSÉRI
25 rue du Grand Pré
10290 Rigny-la-Nonneuse
France
Books in French on Natural Hygiene and the newsletter, *Le Bon
Guide de L'Hygiénisme.*

ORKOS
0033.16460.2111, fax 0033.16460.21.01
toll free in Germany: 0.800.999.8881 fax 0.800.999.888.2
www.orkos.com
info@orkos.com
Huge variety of unprocessed, certified raw, organic foods, both
common and exotic.

RAW FAMILY
P.O. Box 172
Ashland, OR 97520
www.rawfamily.com
Victoria, Igor, Sergei and Valya Boutenko are inspiring examples
for the raw diet. They lead seminars all over the world.

TANGLEWOOD WELLNESS CENTER
6135 Mountaindale Road
Thurmont, MD 21788
301-898-8901
www.tanglewoodwellnesscenter.com
info@TanglewoodWellnessCenter.com

Fasting center and resources on natural hygiene.

HYGIENIC PRACTITIONERS

ARTHUR MICHAEL BAKER MA, NHE
8115 SE Market St
Portland OR 97215
503-774-6611
ArtBaker@HealthCreation.net
http://www.HealthCreation.net

DANA CLARE, BSW, MA, DIP NH
P.O. Box 904
Cooktown
Qld 4871
Australia
Phone: 07-40696967
shankari@bigpond.com

DOUGLAS GRAHAM DC
609 N. Jade Dr
Key Largo, FL 33037 USA
305-743-8882
foodnsport@aol.com
www.doctorgraham.cc

ROZALIND GRUBEN, AHSI, RSA
1 Cassidy Place, New Town Road
Storrington,West Sussex, RH20 4EY, England
Tel/Fax (0) 1903 746572
healthyunlimited@aol.com

DAVID KLEIN, BS, N ED
Living Nutrition Magazine
Colitis & Crohn's Health Recovery Services
PO Box 256 Sebastopol, CA 95473 USA
707-829-0362
dave@livingnutrition.com
http://www.livingnutrition.com

ROBERT SNIADACH, DC
School of Natural Hygiene
1103 Collinwood West Drive
Austin, TX 78753
512-835-1364
rwsniadach@transformationinst.com
www.transformationinst.com

RAY TANNER, DIP NH
9 Balyata Ave., Caringbah, NSW 2229 Australia
Phone: 02-95441553

V VIRGINIA VETRANO, DC, MD
The Rest of Your Life Health School & Retreat
PO Box 102
Barksdale, TX 78828 USA
830.234.3499
vvvetrano@hilconet.com
http://vetrano.cjb.net

SELECTED BIBLIOGRAPHY

JOE ALEXANDER, *Blatant Raw-Foodist Propaganda* (Blue Dolphin, 1990)

T.C. FRY
- *The Myth of Medicine* (Life Science, 1975)
- *Program for Dynamic Health* (Natural Hygiene Press, 1974)

ESSIE HONIBAL AND T C FRY, *I Live on Fruit* (Health Excellence Systems, 1991)

A T HOVANNESSIAN, *Raw Eating* (Hallelujah Acres, 2000)

JULIANO, *Raw: The Uncook Book* (Regan Books, 1999)

FRANZ KONZ, *Der Große Gesundheits-Konz* (Bund Für Gesundheit, 2000)

STEVE MEYEROWITZ, *Sprouts: the Miracle Food* (Sproutman Publications, 1990)

ALBERT MOSSÉRI
- *À la Recherche d'une Santé Parfaite* (Édition Aquarius, 1998)
- *L'homme, le Singe, et le Paradis* (Courrier du Livre, 1990)
- *L'Hygiénisme, Petit Guide du Débutant* (Les Hygiénistes, 1995)
- *Le Jeûne, Meilleur Remède de la Nature* (Les Hygiénistes, 1994)
- *Mangez Nature, Santé Nature, Tome 1 & 2* (Les Hygiénistes, 1992)
- *La Nourriture Idéale et les Combinaisons Simplifiées* (Courrier du Livre, 1976)
- *La Nutrition Hygiéniste* (Éditions Aquarius, 2001)

PAUL NISON, *The Raw Life* (343 Publishing, 2000)

FRÉDÉRIC PATENAUDE
- *The Sunfood Cuisine* (Genesis 1:29, 2002)
- *Just Eat An Apple* Magazine, Vol. 2 #1-3 (Raw Vegan, 2002)

HERBERT SHELTON
- *Food Combining Made Easy* (Willow Publishing, 1982)
- *Orthobionomics* (American Natural Hygiene Society, 1994)
- *The Science and Fine Art of Food and Nutrition* (American Natural Hygiene Society, 1996)
- *Superior Nutrition* (Willow Publishing, 1994)

DAVID WOLFE, *The Sunfood Diet Success System* (Maul Bros, 2000)

GEORGE B SCHALLER, *The Year of the Gorilla* (University of Chicago Press, 1997)

DOUGLAS N GRAHAM, DC
- *Grain Damage* (Self-published, 1998)
- *Nutrition and Athletic Performance* (Self-published, 1999)

ROBERT YOUNG, PH.D., *Sick and Tired? Reclaim Your Inner Terrain* (Woodland Publishing, 2000)

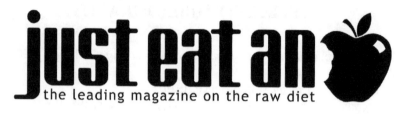

just eat an 🍎

the leading magazine on the raw diet

- RAW DIET
- NATURAL HYGIENE
- VEGETARIANISM

- RADICAL ECOLOGY
- ALTERNATIVE LIFESTYLE
- CONTROVERSIES

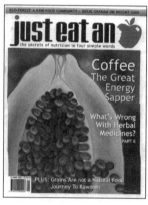

"After reading your magazine, I got totally motivated and inspired to go back to a raw diet."
Shawn Katz , Hove, England

"Thank you for your magazine that I received in the mail last week. To my sheer amazement, within weeks of giving up all animal and processed food, my asthma just stopped!"
Angela Jackson, Amsterdam, Netherland

"Your magazine is growing on me more and more each time that I read (devour) it. I can, it's raw!"
Theresa Taylor, Las Vegas, Nevada

Just Eat An Apple is an alternative diet and health magazine for those interested in raw foodism, vegetarianism, Natural Hygiene and alternative lifestyles. We regularly address what constitutes the raw food diet — an ongoing inquiry and controversy. We spotlight specific foods and relate news from the worldwide, raw food scene; testimonials; ecology; organic farming; and medical and dietary exposés.

Each issue also contains raw vegan recipes, astonishing letters to the editor, questions and answers, and articles written by a wide range of experts from all over the world including: American raw hygienist, Dr. Doug Graham; elder raw hygienic laureate, Albert Mosséri of France; authors, chefs, networkers and raw coaches

Karen Knowler and Shazzie from the UK; editor, researcher and translator, Frederic Patenaude; and serious readers and regular contributors from around the world. Filled with impossible to find information- such as exclusive translations of French and German raw masterpieces, useful contacts, inspiring articles, recipes, interviews and in-depth features, **Just Eat An Apple** is the leading magazine on the raw diet. It is also the networking magazine of the raw vegan community, with three pages of contacts, free classifieds for subscribers, a listing of international events, and intriguing ads from the emerging raw trade.

Just Eat An Apple has subscribers in over 30 countries. First released in August, 1998 as a small, bi-monthly newsletter out of California, JEAA has matured in content and has recently expanded in length and format. Now it is a professionally edited and designed, 48- page, quarterly journal with a full color cover. It will appeal to everyone interested in cutting edge information on health and nutrition.

Visit our website at:
www.justeatanapple.com

TO ORDER, PLEASE USE THE ORDER FORM ON THE NEXT PAGE.

QUICK ORDER FORM

<u>Online Orders:</u> www.rawvegan.com or info@rawvegan.com

<u>Postal Orders:</u> See below.

Please send me: *(All prices US $ and postpaid unless noted)*

___ copies of the book, *The Raw Secrets,* at $14.95 each. (In the USA and Canada, please add $5 shipping for one book and $3 for each additional book. For other countries, add $8 shipping for one book and $5 for each additional book.)

___ 1 year (4 issues) of the magazine, *Just Eat An Apple.* In the USA and Canada: $24, Other countries $36

___ 2 years (8 issues) of the magazine, *Just Eat An Apple.* In the USA and Canada: $42. Other countries: $62

___ sample copies of the magazine *Just Eat An Apple.* USA and Canada: $9. Other Countries: $11

___ booklets, *Raw Soups.* USA and Canada: $7. Other countries: $10

Name: _____

Address: _____

City: _____ State/Province: _____

Postal Code: _____ Country: _____

Telephone: _____ E-mail: _____

Payment (in US Funds): ❏ Check ❏ Money Order ❏ Credit Card:
❏ Visa ❏ MasterCard ❏ American Express

Card Number: _____

Name on card: _____ Exp. date: _____/_____

Send your order to:

Raw Vegan
6595 St-Hubert, CP 59053
Montreal (Quebec)
H2S 3P5, Canada

Comments:_____

_____

_____

_____

QUICK ORDER FORM

<u>Online Orders:</u> www.rawvegan.com or info@rawvegan.com

<u>Postal Orders:</u> See below.

Please send me: *(All prices US $ and postpaid unless noted)*

___ copies of the book, *The Raw Secrets,* at $14.95 each. (In the USA and Canada, please add $5 shipping for one book and $3 for each additional book. For other countries, add $8 shipping for one book and $5 for each additional book.)
___ 1 year (4 issues) of the magazine, *Just Eat An Apple.* In the USA and Canada: $24, Other countries $36
___ 2 years (8 issues) of the magazine, *Just Eat An Apple.* In the USA and Canada: $42. Other countries: $62
___ sample copies of the magazine *Just Eat An Apple.* USA and Canada: $9. Other Countries: $11
___ booklets, *Raw Soups.* USA and Canada: $7. Other countries: $10

Name: _____
Address: _____
City: _____ State/Province: _____
Postal Code: _____ Country: _____
Telephone: _____ E-mail: _____

Payment (in US Funds): ❐ Check ❐ Money Order ❐ Credit Card:
❐ Visa ❐ MasterCard ❐ American Express
Card Number: _____
Name on card: _____ Exp. date: _____/_____

Send your order to:

Raw Vegan
6595 St-Hubert, CP 59053
Montreal (Quebec)
H2S 3P5, Canada

Comments:_____
_____
_____
_____

QUICK ORDER FORM

<u>Online Orders:</u> www.rawvegan.com or info@rawvegan.com

<u>Postal Orders:</u> See below.

Please send me: *(All prices US $ and postpaid)*

___ copies of the book, *The Raw Secrets*, at $14.95 each. (In the USA and Canada, please add $5 shipping for one book and $3 for each additional book. For other countries, add $8 shipping for one book and $5 for each additional book.)

___ 1 year (4 issues) of the magazine, *Just Eat An Apple.* In the USA and Canada: $24, Other countries $36

___ 2 years (8 issues) of the magazine, *Just Eat An Apple.* In the USA and Canada: $42. Other countries: $62

___ sample copies of the magazine *Just Eat An Apple.* USA and Canada: $9. Other Countries: $11

___ booklets, *Raw Soups.* USA and Canada: $7. Other countries: $10

Name: _____

Address: _____

City: _____ State/Province: _____

Postal Code: _____ Country: _____

Telephone: _____ E-mail: _____

Payment (in US Funds): ❏ Check ❏ Money Order ❏ Credit Card:
❏ Visa ❏ MasterCard ❏ American Express

Card Number: _____

Name on card: _____ Exp. date: _____/_____

Send your order to:

Raw Vegan
6595 St-Hubert, CP 59053
Montreal (Quebec)
H2S 3P5, Canada

Comments:_____
_____
_____
_____

For more information on the *raw vegan diet*, to get in contact with other raw-foodists, and to stay abreast of some of the latest breakthroughs in the field,

VISIT OUR WEBSITE:

www.rawvegan.com

ABOUT THE AUTHOR

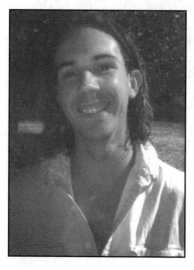

Frédéric Patenaude (b. 1976) edits *Just Eat An Apple*, an international magazine on the raw diet, and leads the publishing company, *Raw Vegan* . He founded *rawvegan.com,* an online resource for raw-foodists and vegetarians and authored the raw recipe book, *The Sunfood Cuisine.* He translates Albert Mosséri's works on Natural Hygiene into English.

A linguist, he speaks French, English, Spanish, Portuguese and German and currently studies Russian. With his many tongues, he translate writings from around the globe for *Just Eat An Apple* and his books and to help build an international network of raw eaters.

He travels, plays classical guitar, cracks jokes and keeps his friend, Andrew, busy and off the street. He lives in Montreal, Canada.

CONSULTATIONS

The author gives affordable consultations by phone. For straight talk and practical advice about eating raw and eating well, write him (see below).

CONTACT

Send your comments, testimonials, questions, e-mail and inquiries to: frederic@rawvegan.com

or write to:

Frédéric Patenaude
6595 St-Hubert, CP 59053
Montreal (Quebec)
H2S 3P5, Canada